Ethics in Reproductive and Perinatal Medicine

CARSON STRONG

Ethics in Reproductive
and Perinatal
Medicine

A NEW FRAMEWORK

Yale University Press
New Haven & London

To my teachers of years long past, especially Lillene Matlock, Eugene Covert, Bill Richards, James Nersoyan, Jim Cornman, and Richard Warner

Set in Sabon type by Keystone Typesetting, Inc., Orwigsburg, Pennsylvania. Printed in the United States of America.

Library of Congress Cataloging-in-Publication Data
Strong, Carson.
    Ethics in reproductive and perinatal medicine : a new framework / Carson Strong.
        p.   cm.
    Includes bibliographical references and index.
    ISBN 0-300-06832-8 (alk. paper)
    1. Human reproductive technology — Moral and ethical aspects.
    2. Perinatology — Moral and ethical aspects.   I. Title.
    [DNLM: 1. Ethics, Medical.   2. Reproduction.   WQ 21 S923e   1997]
    RG133.5.S77   1997
    174'.25 — dc20
    DNLM/DLC
    for Library of Congress   96-18957
                                                                       CIP

A catalogue record for this book is available from the British Library.

The paper in this book meets the guidelines for permanence and durability of the Committee on Production Guidelines for Book Longevity of the Council on Library Resources.

10   9   8   7   6   5   4   3   2   1

Contents

Acknowledgments

This book arises from many years of research, writing, and lecturing on ethical issues in reproductive and perinatal medicine. Along the way, I benefited greatly from the help of colleagues. I am especially grateful for the support given by many faculty physicians in the Department of Obstetrics and Gynecology at the University of Tennessee, Memphis. By encouraging me to participate in the teaching activities of their department, and by openly discussing with me cases raising difficult ethical problems, they enabled me to gain clinical experience that was exceedingly valuable in writing this book. Among these many supporters, a special debt of gratitude is owed to Doug Anderson, Jay Schinfeld, John Dacus, and Guy Photopulos.

Support for this book also was provided by a Summer Stipend from the National Endowment for the Humanities. This grant allowed me to set aside a period of time early in the project for literature searches and reading. The library staff of the Cecil C. Humphreys School of Law at the University of Memphis provided invaluable assistance during the grant period and the following years. Howard Bailey deserves special thanks for helping me navigate the law library.

I also have been fortunate in having had the opportunity to present early versions of parts of this book to various audiences and to benefit from their comments. I am especially indebted to the Society for Health and Human

Values for inviting me to make presentations and providing the opportunity for informal discussions with colleagues. In addition, thanks are owed to the National Advisory Board on Ethics in Reproduction for inviting me to be a member of its Working Group. The meetings of this group have been a valuable source of information and ideas relevant to the book.

Several persons gave significant help by critiquing early drafts of parts of the book. Rosemarie Tong and John Robertson read Chapter 2, Bonnie Steinbock reviewed Chapter 3, and Al Jonsen critiqued Chapter 4. As I had expected, all of them provided insightful comments that helped improve the book. The anonymous reviewers for Yale University Press also made a number of suggestions resulting in needed revisions.

Introduction

Science is moving forward rapidly in reproductive and perinatal medicine. For example, the Human Genome Project is producing a wealth of new information, much of which bears on human reproduction. Already, genes have been identified that cause a number of significant human diseases. Advances in prenatal testing, such as chorionic villus sampling coupled with new and forthcoming genetic tests, are increasing the ability of obstetricians to detect fetal genetic diseases early in pregnancy. Moreover, we are beginning to see the genetic testing of human preembryos and the use of such tests in selecting preembryos for reproduction. The technology of assisted reproduction for infertile couples also is progressing rapidly. In vitro fertilization clinics have proliferated since the birth of the first "test-tube baby" in 1978. Techniques for freezing preembryos have become a standard part of in vitro fertilization programs. Freezing not only permits storage of preembryos for subsequent use by the infertile couple but also facilitates other activities, such as transferring them to a surrogate's uterus, donating them to other infertile couples, and doing research on them. Where genetics and the technologies of assisted reproduction overlap, the future holds the possibility of profound scientific advances. With further developments in gene therapy and the science of genetic manipulation, it might one day be possible to insert and delete parts of chromosomes in human preembryos. Such developments would increase our ability not only to prevent genetic diseases but also to manipulate the genetic make-up of our offspring in yet unseen ways.

These and other scientific advances in reproductive and perinatal medicine are producing a bewildering array of ethical questions. What limits, if any, should be placed on attempts to control the genetic make-up of our children? What restrictions, if any, should we put on methods of assisted reproduction such as ovum donation and surrogate motherhood? To what stage of development should preembryos be kept alive in the laboratory for research purposes? How should a gynecologist respond when a couple requests an abortion in order to select the sex or other nondisease characteristics of their offspring? Is it ethical for physicians to provide artificial insemination to single women? Is it permissible to perform cesarean section against the wishes of a woman for the sake of her fetus? Such questions are rife with controversy, evoking responses ranging from awe and excitement to deep concern. How these issues are handled not only affects the individuals involved in specific cases but can have far-reaching consequences for humankind.

When we consider this array of issues, we see that a considerable number of ethical *values* have a bearing on the decisions to be made. To illustrate this plurality of values, let us briefly consider some of the prominent ones. Reproductive freedom is one of the central values. When we ask, for example, whether we should permit ovum donation to postmenopausal women, we are asking whether we should limit the freedom of persons to engage in this type of reproductive activity. Also, the well-being of the procreators, or potential procreators, is an important consideration, as is the well-being of offspring who would be brought into existence. Respect for life is another important value. The ethics of various actions we might take toward nascent human life, such as discarding preembryos or aborting fetuses, directly depends on the degree of respect that we should give to life at such stages of development. In addition, the well-being of third-party collaborators in assisted reproduction is pertinent. To illustrate: one of the objections to surrogate motherhood is the risk of psychological harm to the surrogate that might be caused by separation from an infant to whom she has become emotionally attached. Another concern is the well-being of society in the immediate and distant future; if new reproductive technologies would help bring about a society in which there is less suffering from infertility and genetic diseases, that would be an important reason to pursue those technologies. Furthermore, preserving autonomy for persons in future generations is an important factor; the possibility of modifying human beings raises the specter of increased control of some persons by others. From another perspective, feminist writers are concerned about whether advances in reproductive technology will increase or decrease the control that women have over their bodies and lives. Considerations of justice are involved, as well. For example, if there is a right to health care, should it include a right to treatment of infertility? How should limited resources be allocated? Yet another important value is scientific freedom. Some governments that have restricted research involving human preembryos, for example, have been criticized for infringing the freedom of scientific investigators.[1] These values are not intended as an exhaustive list, nor is there any special significance to the order in which I have mentioned them. The important point is that *multiple* ethical considerations are relevant to the task of resolving ethical issues in reproductive and perinatal medicine.

In addition, the value *conflicts* involved in these issues are varied and often complex. For any given issue, a particular policy for resolving the issue might tend to support several values, in varying degrees. It might also tend to thwart a number of other values. An alternative policy for resolving the issue might tend to support and thwart different sets of values, in yet different degrees. There might be a number of possible policies for resolving the issue, each having its own distinctive potential for affecting relevant values, so that the selection of a policy involves complicated value judgments.

Not only are the value conflicts complex, but they often include a conflict between the interests of procreators and the interests of their offspring. For example, assisted reproduction sometimes involves new types of family arrangements, such as ovum donation from a sister, who is thus both the social aunt and genetic mother of the child. In deciding whether such assisted reproduction is a good thing, we are led to ask whether these unusual arrangements will result in interpersonal tensions in the family that interfere with the child's well-being. There is a concern that reproductive freedom might be in conflict with the interests of the child in such cases. To consider another example, aggressive treatment for fetuses with serious malformations often involves procedures that pose risks to the pregnant woman. Thus, decisions about whether aggressive treatment is warranted must take into account any conflicts that might exist between the well-being of the pregnant woman and the well-being of the fetus. Resolving issues in reproductive and perinatal medicine therefore requires judgments about how much weight should be given to the interests of procreators and offspring. This does not imply that decisions should consider only these interests, for additional values usually are at stake. However, weighing the interests of procreators and offspring is almost always an important part of the complex problem of resolving these issues.

The Need for an Ethical Framework

To obtain justifiable resolutions of these complex issues, it is necessary to have an ethical framework. Science alone cannot resolve these questions.

Their resolution involves value choices, not purely technical decisions. It requires weighing the conflicting values and deciding priorities.

We need a framework in part because we are unsure how we should weigh the conflicting interests of procreators and offspring. Because the issues are so new, we remain unclear about the nature and importance of these interests. Consider reproductive freedom. A presumption in favor of the freedom of autonomous individuals has been widely recognized since John Stuart Mill's classic essay *On Liberty*. This presumption in favor of freedom entails, more specifically, a presumption in favor of reproductive freedom. However, such a presumption does not resolve the many value conflicts we face because these conflicts almost always pose the question of whether the presumption should be overridden. To better understand how we should weigh procreative freedom against other values, we need to address a number of questions. Why should we consider reproductive freedom valuable? Is it solely because freedom in general is valuable, or is there special significance to the fact that the freedom in question is *reproductive*? What meaning and significance do we attach to having children? Similarly, questions need to be addressed concerning the obligations that parents have toward their offspring. If conceiving a human offspring carries with it certain obligations, what are those obligations? Do they change in strength during pregnancy, and if so, in what way?

Another reason we need a framework is that the traditional theories of ethics, such as utilitarianism and contractarian theories, have serious shortcomings. A number of problems could be mentioned, but one of the most serious is the frequent inability of the theories to produce resolutions to specific cases and policy questions. Because of this problem in bridging the gap between theory and case resolution, these theories often provide little practical guidance. Elsewhere I have discussed in detail how utilitarianism and contractarian theories fail in this regard.[2] Others have discussed in greater depth this shortcoming concerning Kantianism.[3] I do not mean to imply that these theories lack worth or that they should be abandoned. On the contrary, each of them is valuable, in part because it identifies certain ethical considerations that must be taken into account in resolving issues. Nevertheless, the inability of traditional theories to provide practical guidance in clinical situations suggests that a new ethical framework is needed.

What would an acceptable ethical framework for reproductive and perinatal medicine be like? Drawing upon the above discussion, I would like to suggest that such a framework should contain at least three components. First, it should explore and assess the significance of reproductive freedom. Although reproductive freedom is one of the central values in these issues, it has not been examined adequately. Second, because the interests of offspring are among the main values, an ethical framework should address the question of the importance to be attached to those interests. Thus, it should put forward a view concerning the moral status of offspring during the preembryonic, embryonic, fetal, and postnatal stages of development and discuss whatever obligations procreators might have during these stages. Third, it should advocate an approach to the problem of assigning priorities to conflicting values. The chosen approach should take into account all relevant ethical considerations, including the plurality of values and the considerations identified by the traditional ethical theories that I mentioned above. The approach also, of course, should provide practical guidance in resolving policy questions and individual cases.

In the many articles and books about reproductive ethics, no author has previously put forward a framework that includes all three of these elements. Two recently published books, John A. Robertson's *Children of Choice* and Laurence B. McCullough and Frank A. Chervenak's *Ethics in Obstetrics and Gynecology*,[4] propose quite different ethical frameworks, but neither satisfies the requirements outlined above. Robertson's framework falls short on two counts. First, although it contains views about the moral standing of pre-embryos and children, it does not provide a systematic account of moral status throughout the periods of preembryonic, embryonic, and fetal development. Second, in addressing conflicting values, Robertson focuses on the social policy issue concerning the justification of state interference with procreative freedom. He deals with the problem, which arises in constitutional law, of identifying state interests that are sufficiently compelling to justify such interference. This type of policy-level issue can be contrasted with clinical issues that arise in particular cases. An example would be the question of what recommendations, if any, a physician should make to a pregnant woman when fetal anomalies have been detected. A choice between recommending aggressive or nonaggressive management, for example, involves weighing maternal and fetal interests. Robertson's book does not address such clinical issues, nor is his constitutional-law approach able to deal with the value conflicts that arise in the clinical setting.

There also are two main ways in which the framework presented by McCullough and Chervenak falls short of these requirements. First, their book contains little or no exploration of the importance of procreative freedom and reasons for valuing it. Second, although they discuss the weighing of conflicting values, they do so primarily in the context of clinical issues. With regard to policy-level ethical issues of the sort Robertson examines, McCullough and Chervenak have relatively little to say, and they make no attempt to formulate an explicit approach to the weighing of values in the context of such social issues.[5]

Thus, the two books contrast sharply: Robertson's framework is not capable of addressing clinical issues, while McCullough and Chervenak's has little to say about policy-level issues. Taken together, they present a dichotomy between the two types of issues. However, there is no need to accept such a dichotomy. The framework that I shall put forward in this book seeks to address both policy-level *and* clinical issues.

Preview of the Book

In Part 1, I attempt to provide an ethical framework containing the three components identified above. In Chapter 1, I address the question of why *freedom to procreate* should be considered valuable. I do this by examining some reasons why procreating might be personally significant to individuals. In addition to discussing what is involved in procreative freedom, I take up the question of whether there is a *right* to reproduce and argue that there is indeed such a right. In Chapter 2, I consider why *freedom not to procreate* should be considered valuable, drawing upon two types of sources. The first is U.S. Supreme Court cases concerning the constitutional right to freedom from state intrusion in making procreative decisions, as well as the extensive legal literature concerning those cases. The second is the writings of feminists who have addressed this topic. I put forward a view concerning the importance of freedom not to procreate that takes into account both the legal and feminist literature.

In Chapter 3, I discuss the moral status of offspring during various stages of gestation. A number of views have been put forward and an enormous amount has been written on this subject. Trying to add something new is a daunting task. Yet, a significant feature of this chapter is the articulation and defense of a view that has not been put forward by others. This view draws upon the idea, held widely but not universally, that the moral standing of the fetus becomes progressively stronger as fetal development proceeds. One of the main contributions of this chapter — and of the book as a whole — is the formulation of this idea in a new and distinctive way. I also maintain that the strength of parental obligations can be affected by the fetus's moral standing. Further implications of my view concerning progressively greater moral standing are explored in Part 2 by applying it to issues involving different stages of gestation.

In Chapter 4, I address the problem of assigning priorities to conflicting ethical values. Four main approaches are contrasted. After considering the pros and cons of each approach, I defend one of them, a version of casuistic reasoning. The reader who would like a "sneak preview" of the ethical framework developed in Part 1 can turn to the end of Chapter 4, where a summary is provided. My conclusion that this framework is justifiable is tentative, however. A further test of its acceptability comes in Part 2 when we consider the degree to which it is helpful in resolving the issues addressed.

In Part 2, I bring the framework to bear upon some of the main ethical issues in reproductive and perinatal medicine. For each issue, I attempt to identify the main ethical views, assess their pros and cons, and defend a view. The assessment of opposing views draws upon the framework of Part 1, using its conclusions concerning the significance of reproductive freedom and the moral status of offspring. Chapter 5 explores issues arising from new family arrangements made possible by techniques for assisted reproduction. Topics addressed include donor insemination for single women, ovum donation for "older" women, and surrogate motherhood. Chapter 6 deals with issues concerning the manipulation of preembryos, including creating, freezing, transferring, donating, and discarding them. It also addresses research on preembryos and disposition of preembryos following divorce. In Chapter 7, I discuss issues in reproductive genetics, focusing on topics that involve the selection of offspring characteristics. Specifically, I discuss prenatal testing for "minor" diseases and nondisease characteristics, preimplantation genetic testing, and the selection of gamete donors to enhance the characteristics of offspring. Chapter 8 turns to decisions following detection of fetal anomalies, and it focuses on the question of what recommendations, if any, the physician should make to the pregnant woman. Finally, the topic of coercive interventions during pregnancy, performed for the sake of the fetus, is covered in Chapter 9.

Part 2 is not intended to be a comprehensive study of *all* issues in reproductive and perinatal medicine. Space limitations dictated that some important issues be omitted. Several considerations guided my choice of topics to be covered. First, the chapters collectively should address the main conceptual issues that arise in reproductive and perinatal ethics. I suggest that these conceptual issues include the following: how reasons for valuing procreative freedom have a bearing on the resolution of issues; how conflicts between procreative freedom and other values, including the interests of offspring, should be resolved; the reasons for and against modifying our offspring through genetic technology; and how the moral standing of offspring might vary at different stages of gestation. Second, the topics should be interesting to the reader. Third, the topics should be useful for illustrating the main points of the ethical framework developed in Part 1.

Parts 1 and 2 are integrated in several ways. Development of the framework in Part 1 provides principles and concepts for analyzing the issues in Part 2. Conversely, discussion of the issues illustrates the implications of the framework. The book concludes with a brief epilogue discussing main ways in which the framework proves useful in addressing the issues.

Although this book is subtitled "A New Framework," I acknowledge that the framework I set forth is not entirely new. After all, many have come before me, and my work in large part is a synthesis. What is new is the identification of the main components of an ethical framework for reproductive and perinatal medicine and the setting forth of those components in some detail. Also, something new is said about each of these components. In particular, I attempt to advance the debate in each of these areas: the importance and meaning of reproductive freedom; the moral status of offspring during various stages of prenatal development; and the explication and defense of casuistry as a method of assigning priorities to conflicting values. I also acknowledge that what I say herein is certainly not the final word. Rather, it is my hope that this book will convince the reader that an explicit framework for addressing reproductive and perinatal ethics is useful, even necessary, and that increased attention should be paid to the question of what form such a framework should take.

PART I

An Ethical Framework

I

Is There a Right to Reproduce?

In 1935, Oklahoma passed a law called the Habitual Criminal Sterilization Act. This statute, which arose from the eugenics movement, was based on the view that criminal tendencies can be genetically transmitted to offspring. After the third felony conviction, a prisoner was classified as a "habitual offender" and could be brought to court by the state attorney general to determine whether sterilization, by vasectomy for males and salpingectomy for females, should be performed. If the prisoner could be sterilized "without detriment to his or her general health," the court was required to authorize the sterilization.[1]

Another example from the history of sterilization in America is the case of fifteen-year-old Linda Spitler. In July 1971, Linda's mother petitioned the Circuit Court of DeKalb County, Indiana, to authorize a tubal ligation for her daughter. The petition stated that Linda was "somewhat retarded," although she attended public school and had been promoted each year with her class. It pointed out that Linda had been associating with "older youth or young men" and had stayed overnight with them on several occasions. Given this behavior and her mental retardation, the petition asserted, it would be in Linda's best interests to be sterilized in order "to prevent unfortunate circumstances." Judge Harold D. Stump authorized the sterilization without seeking a professional assessment of Linda's mental and behavioral capacities. Moreover, the decision followed an informal session without advance notice to Linda, appointment of a guardian *ad litem,* or a hearing. Soon afterward the tubal ligation was performed. Linda was unaware of the nature of the procedure, having been told that the purpose was to remove her appendix. Approximately two years later she married Leo Sparkman, and her inability to become pregnant led to her discovery that she had been sterilized.[2]

Quite plainly, the use of sterilization in these examples was wrong for a number of reasons. First, the view that criminal propensities are inheritable has long been discredited. Second, in the Spitler case the use of deception and absence of due process are highly disturbing, as is the strong undercurrent of discrimination against the mentally retarded. Beyond these features, however, a fundamental ethical criticism is that involuntary sterilization is a violation of procreative freedom because it denies persons the ability to make their own decisions about whether to have children and how many to have. This aspect of the examples will be the focus of my discussion.

The main question I want to explore in this chapter is *why* procreative freedom should be valued. Why do we think it is wrong to deprive Linda Spitler — or someone who has been convicted of felonies three times in Oklahoma — of the ability to have children? An easy answer is that freedom in general is valuable, and therefore any type of freedom, including procreative freedom, is valuable. However, I want to explore the matter further. Is procreative freedom valuable simply because it is a type of freedom, or is there special significance in the fact that these decisions are *procreative* ones? A frequently raised question is whether there is a *right* to reproduce.[3] Sometimes it is asserted that there is no such right.[4] The question of how one might defend a right to procreate has received surprisingly little attention, but if there is such a right, we should try to clarify its basis.

Various reasons could be given for the importance of procreation. At a "macro" level, survival of the species depends on it. Similarly, trends in birth rates have an impact on the economic and social well-being of communities and nations. For example, the surge in population during the "baby boom" generation has raised concerns about resources for future health care for the elderly. However, in this book I shall deal with the topic at the "micro" level — the level of individual persons. What is the personal meaning and ethical significance of procreative freedom for individuals?

There are two main components of procreative freedom: freedom to procreate and freedom not to procreate.[5] As we shall see, the reasons for valuing these components are not entirely identical. Therefore, the questions raised will be explored by considering these components separately. This chapter will deal with freedom to procreate, the next chapter with freedom not to procreate. To explore why *freedom* to procreate should be considered important, it is helpful to begin by considering what is meant by *procreation*.

What Is Procreation?

We can think of procreation as involving three main elements, one of which is *begetting* — producing offspring that are genetically one's own.[6] One can beget, of course, by artificial methods such as in vitro fertilization as well as by coitus. The second element is *gestating,* and the third is *rearing* children. Of course, procreators need not participate in all three components. For example, sperm and ovum donors beget without gestating or rearing. Similarly, one can gestate without begetting or rearing, as in the case of a surrogate mother who receives a fertilized ovum from an infertile couple. Thus, the terms *genetic parent, gestational parent,* and *social parent* sometimes are used to distinguish these roles.

One might ask why rearing should be considered part of procreating. After all, the child has been brought into being by the time rearing is undertaken. One commentator states that child rearing is not reproduction, strictly speaking, but suggests that because the role of social parent can be of great importance to persons, decisions to enter or leave that role should be regarded as procreative.[7] The problem with this view is that rearing, as well as entering and leaving the rearing role, sometimes clearly do not constitute procreating. For example, it would seem odd to say that infertile couples become procreators by adopting children and rearing them.

Nevertheless, rearing contributes to the creating of a person, just as begetting and gestating do. Those who rear are instrumental in shaping the unique person that the child becomes. Given this influence, it seems appropriate to include rearing under procreation. But this would imply that whoever heavily influences a child's development should be considered a procreator. We would have to say that the "shaping" provided by influential preachers, boarding school teachers, or older siblings was procreation!

However, we still could say that rearing carried out by those who beget or gestate the child is part of procreating. First, people often desire to beget so that they will have children to rear. In such cases, begetting, gestating, and rearing can be viewed as a continuum of events that make up the overall endeavor of having children. Second, when parents rear a child they have begotten or gestated, their shaping of the child's character and development can be viewed as an extension of their creation of the child. By contrast, the shaping of a child by adoptive parents is not a continuation of their creation of the child but rather a wholly new undertaking. For these reasons, I shall consider rearing to be part of procreating, provided it is the rearing of a child one has begotten or gestated.

A separate question concerns what is involved in freedom to procreate. Two senses of this expression can be distinguished. In the strict sense, it involves only the freedom to choose to procreate. This is the type of freedom involved in the examples at the beginning of this chapter. It includes the freedoms to choose to beget, to gestate, and to raise one's genetic or gestational offspring. In a second and broader sense, the term could be understood to include freedom to make additional decisions associated with one's procreation. For example, a couple might decide to have their preembryos tested genetically prior to uterine transfer. This might be thought of as part of their decision to try to procreate. However, a decision to test is not the same as a decision to try to procreate. Freedom to procreate in this broader sense covers a variety of decisions, such as freedom to choose fetal therapy, midwifery for prenatal care, and birthing methods.[8] Whether certain of these procreative freedoms in the broader sense should be valued and protected to the same degree as freedom to procreate in the strict sense is an important question. For example, in addressing preimplantation genetic testing in Chapter 7, I shall consider freedom to select the genetic characteristics of our children.

Here I shall focus on freedom to procreate in the strict sense. My strategy is to try to understand why this fundamental sense of freedom to procreate is important, and then to use this understanding to address some of the new issues involving freedom to procreate in the broader sense. Moreover, I believe that insights can be gained by focusing especially on a category of procreation commonly referred to as "having a child of one's own," sometimes stated simply as "having a child" or "having children." The expression "having a child of one's own" might be interpreted in several ways, so let me be specific. I am using it to refer to begetting a child whom one rears or helps rear. This, of course, is the common form of procreation, involving parents who raise children who are genetically their own. Certainly, not all procreation fits into this category, but it is an important place to start in considering the personal meaning of procreation for individuals.[9]

Our culture is imbued with the attitude that it is important to have children of one's own. There is no better way to appreciate the intensity and prevalence of this attitude than by considering the emotional response of couples who learn that they are unable to have children of their own because of infertility. Let us briefly consider the nature of this response.

Emotional Reactions to Infertility

Authors with extensive clinical experience in counseling infertile couples have described the psychological and emotional aspects of infertility.[10] Although the response varies from one infertile person to the next, infertility often is perceived as a crisis, a threat to deeply held desires. It is typical for infertile couples to experience a grief response involving one or more features, including shock, denial, anger, guilt, and depression.

The initial reaction usually is psychic shock and surprise. For many people, parenthood is a highly planned event. Having children sometimes is delayed in order to develop careers or carry out other projects. The attempt to have children can follow extended periods of using birth control, based on the conviction that if contraception is not used, pregnancy will occur. Many people are not prepared for the possibility of infertility. Denial is a common reaction at this point. "This can't be happening to me!" they say. Denial allows persons to adjust at their own rate to a perceived loss, and the actual or potential losses are multiple. They include loss of control over important plans, loss of a desired role of biological parent, and loss of status in the eyes of others. Some maintain their denial even after years of unsuccessfully attempting pregnancy. Acknowledgment of infertility often leads to anger over one's plight. Some infertile people experience feelings of guilt. They ask themselves whether they have done something to bring on infertility, and review their past for deeds that might be the cause. Some ask whether God is punishing them for something they have done. Sources of guilt can include premarital sex, use of contraceptives, abortion, impregnation, venereal disease, or extramarital affairs. As hope for genetic offspring diminishes, depression occurs in some cases. This might be associated with fear of abandonment by one's spouse. In women, mood swings can occur with the menstrual cycle: with each onset of menstruation, signaling that pregnancy has not been achieved, the initial response can be sadness or even despair.[11]

Moreover, infertility patients often feel defective and inferior. This sense of inferiority concerning reproductive capacity can extend to similar feelings about one's sexual capacities, desirability, and physical attractiveness. Temporary sexual dysfunction, such as impotence or loss of libido, sometimes occurs. Also, a general loss of self-esteem can occur which adversely affects employment, friendships, and marital relationships.[12]

The various responses described above can lead to increased isolation. It might become uncomfortable to be with friends and relatives who fail to understand the emotional effects of infertility. It might become increasingly painful to associate with those who have babies. Guilt and feelings of inferiority can create a tendency to be secretive about the infertility, leading to withdrawal.[13]

In providing this litany of responses, I do not mean to imply that infertile couples always "go off the deep end." Some do not experience all of these reactions, and some responses are not severe. However, difficulties in coping are common. Much of the clinical literature cited above emphasizes the need of infertile couples for emotional support and counseling from health care providers. These reactions show that the desire to have genetic offspring runs deep. Additional empirical studies support the claim that these desires are widespread.[14] However, the *reasonableness* of considering it important to have genetic offspring is a separate question, one to which we now turn.

Is It Reasonable to Want Children of One's Own?

The comedian Bill Cosby has stated, "In talking to audiences around the country, I have conducted my own Cosby Poll, asking parents, 'Why did you have children when all your other acts were rational?' "[15]

Others have made the same point in earnest, arguing that the desire for genetic offspring is unreasonable. Some maintain that the desire to beget is due to social conditioning arising from pressures on men and women to marry and reproduce.[16] These pressures have been referred to as "the parenthood prescription,"[17] and their existence has been confirmed by a number of studies.[18] There is pressure not only to become a parent but also to have children that are genetically one's own. Judith N. Lasker and Susan Borg asked infertile couples why they persisted with infertility treatments rather than trying to adopt a child.[19] Although a variety of answers were given, a common theme was that the desire to keep trying to have a baby is powerfully reinforced from the outside—from media accounts of "miracle" babies, from other patients who have succeeded, from doctors who recommend in vitro fertilization, and from friends who suggest new methods they have heard about.

It is often noted that the desires of women to beget can be influenced by yet other pressures in our culture.[20] Sex-role stereotyping has been a pervasive feature of our society, and central to this stereotyping is the view that a woman's role should consist mainly in having children and taking care of them. Although parenthood is "prescribed" for all married adults, it is considered to be more important for women than for men. Nancy Felipe Russo refers to this as the "motherhood mandate." She states that "the centrality of motherhood to the definition of the adult female is characterized in the form of a mandate which requires having at least two children and raising them well."[21] From a feminist perspective, this conditioning reflects the values of a male-dominated society. Feminists suggest that it is men rather than women who desire genetic offspring and that the conditioning of women serves to satisfy this male desire.[22]

Michael Bayles has argued that the desire to have genetic offspring is irrational.[23] According to him, the rationality of a desire is ascertained by considering whether one would hold it if all the relevant available information and logic were brought to bear on it. If one would hold it in face of such scrutiny, then it is rational; if one would not hold it, then it is irrational. Bayles asks us to consider the desire to beget in order to raise children that are genetically one's own. Would one desire this if all the information and logic were brought to bear? Bayles claims that one test for answering this question is whether fulfillment of the desire would contribute anything to one's life experience. Specifically, he asks us to consider the difference between rearing one's genetic offspring and rearing a child that is not genetically one's own, in terms of the experiences one would have. Bayles claims that the experiences do not seem to be different, except for the belief that the child is genetically one's own. He then claims that this difference is not important. The argument he gives is that "if the genetic relation were important, it would imply that adoptive parents cannot have as valuable experiences of child rearing as natural parents, which seems false."[24]

Admittedly, for some people the desire to beget is influenced by social conditioning. However, in exploring whether it is *reasonable* to value begetting, the important issue is not whether people are conditioned to value it, but whether reasons can be given to justify valuing it. The psychosocial origins of a desire and its justification are two different things. Similarly, even if the desires of many women to beget are conditioned by traditional attitudes about sex-roles, it does not rule out the possibility that there are good reasons that can be given by a woman to support the belief that begetting is important. Moreover, it is fully consistent with the values of equality and liberty underlying the women's movement to suggest that there are valid reasons supporting the desire to beget. Many feminist writers have positive attitudes toward pregnancy, childbirth, and motherhood, while holding that they should not be considered sufficient, in and of themselves, for a woman's self-fulfillment.[25]

With regard to Bayles's claim that a genetic tie to the children one is raising does not contribute to one's life experiences, we might ask whether there are, in fact, important special experiences associated with it. If there are, then Bayles's assertion that the experiences of adoptive parents are just as valuable as those of biological parents misses the point. What matters, on Bayles's own account of rational desire, is whether there are important experiences arising from the fact of genetic relatedness, not whether they are more or less valuable than other types of experiences.[26] Thus, to respond to Bayles's argument, we must consider whether there are reasons that justify the desire for genetic offspring, including reasons why genetic relatedness can be a source of valuable experiences.

Reasons for Valuing Procreation

Studies have identified a variety of reasons people actually give for having children, some of which seem rather selfish or confused.[27] For example, some people desire children as a way of demonstrating their virility or femininity. The views that underlie such reasons — that virility is central to the worth of a man, and that women must have babies to prove their femininity — are open to challenge. Not only do they reflect traditional sex-role stereotypes, but they overlook ways in which self-esteem can be enhanced other than by propagating. To consider another example, sometimes a child is desired to "save" a shaky marriage. This reason fails to address the causes of the marital problems, and the added stress of raising a child might further strain the marital relationship. By contrast, we want to consider whether there are defensible reasons that can be given for desiring genetic offspring. I suggest that the main reasons that have merit include the following:

PARTICIPATION IN THE CREATION OF A PERSON

A normal outcome of human begetting is the creation of a person, an individual with self-consciousness. Philosophers have regarded self-consciousness with wonder and have asked enduring questions about it: What is the relation between mind and body? How can consciousness arise from the physical matter of the brain? There is irony in the fact that although we have great difficulty answering these questions, we are capable of bringing self-consciousness into existence with relative ease. Each of us who begets an individual who becomes self-conscious participates in the creation of a person. As Joseph Ellin has pointed out, "the idea of 'participation in creation' does seem to have certain metaphysical and spiritual overtones that go beyond mere biological reproduction."[28] Perhaps those who have children usually do not think about procreation in these terms. Yet, this is a reason that can be given to help justify the desire for genetic offspring. The creation of a person might be regarded by some as an important event, in which we participate in the mystery of the creation of self-consciousness.

AFFIRMATION OF MUTUAL LOVE

Intentionally having offspring can be an affirmation of a couple's mutual love and acceptance of each other. It can be a deep expression of acceptance to say to another, in effect, "I want your genes to contribute to the genetic make-up of my offspring." Moreover, in such a context there is often anticipation that the bond between the couple will grow stronger because of common children to whom each has a genetic relationship. To purposefully seek the strengthening of personal bonds in this manner can be a further affirmation of mutual love and acceptance.

CONTRIBUTION TO SEXUAL INTIMACY

The term *intimate* derives from the Latin *intimus,* meaning "innermost." It refers to what is most private or personal. An intimate friend or companion is one with whom personal feelings and private matters are shared. As Jeffrey H. Reiman points out, what constitutes intimacy is not merely the sharing of private information, but a context of *caring* which makes the sharing of personal information significant. As he states, "Necessary to an intimate relationship such as friendship or love is a reciprocal desire to share present and future intense and important experiences together."[29]

It goes without saying that lovemaking is an intimate act. One's body is revealed to the other, as are one's sexual needs and desires. As Reiman puts it: "In sexual intimacy one is literally and symbolically stripped of the ordinary masks that obstruct true sharing of experience. This happens not merely in the nakedness of lovers but even more so in the giving of themselves over to the physical forces in their bodies. In surrendering the ordinary restraints, lovers allow themselves to be what they truly are — at least as bodies — intensely and together."[30] To the extent that the feelings and thoughts of the partners also are shared in a caring context, lovemaking becomes all the more intimate.

Thus, the intimacy that occurs in lovemaking between a man and woman can be described using a cluster of concepts pertaining to physical and psychological sharing: sharing one's privacy; giving oneself; having mutual desires to share important experiences; and having access to the innermost part of the other. In physical terms, the features of sexual intimacy are obvious. The man is inside the woman. A woman opens herself to receiving a man's sperm that comes from within his body. Given a context of mutual caring, it might be asked what could be more intimate.

Yet, even greater intimacy is possible when the couple willingly makes love in a manner that is open to procreation. This added intimacy also has physical and psychological components. The sharing and combining of gametes literally carries physical intimacy a step further, constituting the ultimate union of man and woman. Moreover, the willingness of partners to join in this manner can express a further commitment to one another, a desire to share future important experiences associated with parenting.

It should be self-evident that this procreative intimacy is important to persons. To underscore this point, it is worth noting that the possible loss of this intimacy that might result from the separation of lovemaking and procreation in new reproductive technologies is a matter of great concern to some. Opposition to assisted reproduction such as in vitro fertilization and artificial insemination has been based in part on this potential loss of intimacy.[31]

LINK TO FUTURE PERSONS

In Plato's *Symposium,* Socrates points out three ways in which people attempt to gain immortality — performing great deeds, authorship, and having children. Needless to say, immortality in the sense of personal survival cannot be attained by these methods. However, with regard to having children, a more modest goal of establishing a link to future persons can be achieved. Some might value having such a genetic link, for various reasons: it can be thought of as a personal contribution to the future of the human community and its survival; or it might reflect one's judgment about how one's life counts and how far its influence extends.[32]

Although having offspring can make a contribution to the membership of future generations, the degree to which one thereby secures a link to the future is modest, at best. By having children, one's genes will be passed on and one will be remembered, but this impact will be limited. Perhaps one's children or grandchildren will not reproduce. Even if they do, the genes that are inherited in subsequent generations become reduced in number. By the fifth generation, only one-sixteenth of the originator's genes remain, and in time the percentage becomes minute. Also, remembrance is lost as generations pass. After all, how much do most of us know about our forebears four or five generations back?[33] These observations echo a point made by Plato in the *Symposium,* that the link to the future typically gained through begetting pales in comparison to that which can arise from great deeds or authorship.[34] Moreover, having a genetic tie to future persons cuts both ways. As Bill Cosby puts it: "Poets have said the reason to have children is to give yourself immortality; and I must admit I did ask God to give me a son because I wanted someone to carry on the family name. Well, God did just that and I now confess that there have been times when I've told my son not to reveal who he is."[35] Nevertheless, even those who recognize that a link to future persons through children is likely to be modest might consider it important to have that link.

EXPERIENCE OF PREGNANCY AND CHILDBIRTH

For women, having children can be meaningful in part because it involves experiences associated with pregnancy and childbirth. It should be noted, of course, that many women do not find such experiences desirable.

Discomforts can be significant and include nausea, back pain, and feeling tired. There can be negative psychological experiences, including anxiety about the baby's health, fear of death, irritability, insomnia, mood swings, and "maternity blues." Despite the negatives, some women do find the experience on balance to be valuable. One of the satisfactions sometimes experienced by pregnant women is increased attention or esteem from others. Pregnant women frequently are treated with deference and respect, and husbands often respond with increased tenderness and consideration. Another reported satisfaction is an experience of joy immediately after the birth of the child.

No doubt, the responses toward pregnant women and the satisfactions women derive from pregnancy sometimes are manifestations of traditional sex-role stereotyping and social conditioning. Others may respond favorably and women may feel good about being pregnant because they are fulfilling what is still widely viewed as their central role. However, additional factors can foster desirable experiences associated with pregnancy. A pregnant woman might experience enhanced self-esteem from the fact that pregnancy, particularly a first pregnancy, can signify a step toward maturity. I do not mean to imply that pregnancy or parenting is necessary for maturity, but the perception that pregnancy can sometimes contribute to maturity seems well founded. For example, a woman's perceived responsibilities toward her fetus might have a maturing effect. Pregnancy is viewed by some as a learning experience that contributes to self-enrichment and development. Also, the personal satisfaction that can be derived from altruistic behavior should not be overlooked, since pregnancy can involve significant sacrifices for the sake of the fetus. Given these considerations, there seem to be valid reasons for finding the experience of pregnancy and childbirth personally meaningful.

EXPERIENCE OF CHILD REARING

Having children of one's own can be valued in part because it involves experiences associated with rearing. Of course, some people do not enjoy being with children, much less raising them. Raising children is a long and demanding process requiring time, energy, and money. Psychological stress and anxiety are common features. Despite these disadvantages, many people find the experience of raising children highly rewarding. Children provide stimulation and entertainment. Many parents gain a sense of accomplishment and pleasure from helping and watching children develop skills and talents. A child can be not only enjoyable company but someone with whom to share love. In addition, people who feel a need to be altruistic can find in child rearing a way to be giving and caring.

An added significance arises from raising children who are genetically one's own. In this situation, one participates even more fully in the creation of a person. Not only does one help shape personality and develop skills, but one has participated in the physical coming into being of the individual. Furthermore, there is often a family resemblance to at least one of the parents. In some cases this resemblance can serve as a constant reminder of the special significance the child has as an expression of love the parents have for each other. For reasons such as these, raising one's own children can involve important experiences that differ from, without necessarily being more valuable than, those associated with rearing adopted children.

We have identified a number of reasons why having children of one's own can be meaningful to persons. These reasons are not meant to be exhaustive, but they are sufficient to show that procreating can be important. Also, I do not mean to imply that one *ought* to desire genetic offspring, but only that the desire can be justified. Although some feminists have claimed that it is men primarily who desire to have genetic offspring, I would point out that all of the reasons stated above can plausibly be given by women.

These reasons also suggest that procreating can contribute to one's self-identity, one's sense of who one is. For example, whether one has helped create another person can be part of one's self-identity. Similarly, whether one has gestated, is a rearing parent, or has a certain kind of link to the future can be part of one's sense of who one is. Of course, for some these factors might not have a great bearing on self-identity, but for others they can be important. The reasons identified also suggest that procreating can be important to self-fulfillment. It permits marital love to be enriched and marital intimacy to be deepened. For some, bearing or raising children of one's own contributes to personal fulfillment. I would like to suggest that these considerations help explain, at least partially, the grief response of infertile couples. Among other things, infertility is a threat to self-identity and self-fulfillment.

The reasons identified show why the desire to have children of one's own can be rational. They also help explain why *freedom* to procreate should be valued; namely, because procreation can be important to persons in the ways discussed above, including contributing to self-identity and self-fulfillment.

A Right to Reproduce

To address the question of whether there is a right to reproduce, we need to consider what is involved in having a right. Often rights are characterized as a type of *claim*. A widely quoted account is that of Joel Feinberg, who points out that to have a moral right is to have a claim the recognition of which is called for by moral principles. To have a claim, in turn, is to have a case meriting consideration, to have grounds that put one in a position to demand one's due.[36]

Furthermore, it is customary to distinguish between negative and positive rights. Negative rights are valid claims to *noninterference* with activities or states of affairs. An important feature of negative rights is that interference with the right is justifiable only if there is a sufficiently weighty moral reason supporting the interference.[37] This implies that negative rights are prima facie claims. They constitute a presumption that others should avoid interference, but in special circumstances such presumptions can be overridden by other moral concerns. Positive rights are valid claims to be *provided* with something by others. For example, if infertile couples have a right to be provided in vitro fertilization procedures, at state expense if necessary, that right would be a positive one. Whether there is such a right is a matter of debate.[38]

In this chapter we are concerned primarily with negative rights. The sterilization examples at the beginning of the chapter raised the question of whether there is a negative right to reproduce. Furthermore, because positive rights require more of others than mere noninterference, their justification is more difficult and seemingly more complex than that of negative rights. Therefore, we shall focus for now on the less formidable question of whether there is a negative right to reproduce.

It might be thought that the language of rights leads to difficulties when applied to procreation. The bearers of rights are usually considered to be individuals, but procreation normally requires a male and a female (putting aside cloning and parthenogenesis). The idea that a person has a right to do something that an individual cannot do alone has seemed puzzling to some. For example, in discussing the right to procreate, Leon Kass asks, "Whose right is it, a woman's or a couple's?"[39] If there is a right to reproduce, neither would be a satisfactory answer. It would not make sense to restrict the right to women, given that interferences with procreative freedom can occur to men and women alike. Also, one need not make procreative rights a special case by saying that they are possessed by couples, not individuals. To be sure, interferences with procreative freedom can be felt by both members of a couple, but in such cases we can say that there is an interference with the procreative freedom of each. Moreover, interferences sometimes affect an individual, not a couple. Consider a forced sterilization of a single person who afterward is celibate. For these reasons, the fact that procreation requires two persons does not seem to create special obstacles to talking about rights.

Another objection is that too much attention is given to discussions about rights. There is concern that a preoccupation with rights tends to make us overlook other important aspects of moral life. I agree that there are other important concepts in moral discourse, including harms, benefits, responsibilities, virtues, and features of human relationships such as caring and fidelity. Moreover, a plurality of values are relevant to ethical issues in human reproduction, as I pointed out in the Introduction and will further elaborate upon in Chapter 4. However, the objection in question sometimes is stated too forcefully, to the point of disparaging almost any effort to discuss rights.[40] I want to avoid the two extremes of focusing exclusively on rights and avoiding discussion of rights. The concept of rights is important in reproductive and perinatal ethics in part because a number of issues arise concerning whether the state should restrict individual liberties. This book would be seriously deficient if it failed to address rights.

We need to ask what kind of moral reason for noninterference there must be in order for one to have a negative right. This question can be answered by drawing upon the somewhat vague but nevertheless helpful Kantian notion of treating others as ends in themselves. The concept of rights is closely aligned to Kantian, as opposed to consequentialist, ethical theory; violating someone's rights is an inherently wrong-making feature of an action regardless of its consequences. Moral rights go hand in hand with the Kantian concept of respect for persons, the idea that there are ways of treating persons that are inconsistent with the degree of consideration they deserve as members of the moral community.[41] I would like to suggest that this close relationship between moral rights and respect for persons can be expressed as follows: If an interference would constitute treating a person as a mere means and not as an end in himself, then we have a reason of the relevant kind for saying that the person has a moral right to be free from that interference.

Given the features of rights discussed above, at least two important considerations are pertinent to deciding whether a particular freedom from interference can be claimed as a matter of right. Let us see how these considerations apply to the question of whether there is a right to reproduce.

The primary consideration is whether the noninterference is a requirement of treating persons as ends in themselves, as having the dignity and full moral standing that is due to them. We have seen that procreating can be important to self-identity and self-fulfillment. To deprive persons of the capacity to reproduce can significantly alter self-identity and diminish potential for self-fulfillment. Intentionally to treat individuals in ways that are likely to cause such losses would constitute a failure to accord them the full respect they deserve as persons. In addition, the psychological responses to infertility indicate that many persons associate the capacity to procreate with self-worth and normalcy. Given these social attitudes, regardless of whether they are rationally grounded, to interfere with procreative capacity can be a denigration of persons. When interferences involve bodily intrusions, as in sterilizations, there is an added disrespect in the form of a violation of the bodily integrity of persons.

A second consideration is whether there are examples in which our moral intuitions suggest that interference with the freedom in question is wrong. When a particular freedom is not a matter of right, then no special reason is needed to justify an interference. Therefore, if we can identify examples in which our intuitions tell us that the interference is wrong, and in which the wrongness arises in significant part precisely from the interference itself, then that suggests that special reasons *are* needed to justify that type of interference (and that such special reasons are absent in the cases in question). Admittedly, different people sometimes have opposing intuitions about examples. Nevertheless, our firm intuitions can constitute a strong presumption concerning the rightness or wrongness of actions.

Let us consider the examples discussed at the beginning of this chapter. With regard to the Oklahoma habitual criminal law, our intuitions tell us that the proposed forced sterilizations would be wrong. Not only was the eugenic theory underlying the law false, but forced sterilization is highly intrusive and harmful.[42] Similarly, it is clear that the sterilization of Linda Spitler was wrong. Not only was the court order issued in a manner that seemed to lack concern for her interests, but her ability to have children of her own was taken away. Thus, our intuitions about these examples support the view that special reasons *are* needed in order to justify interferences with the freedom to procreate. These two considerations taken together provide strong support for the view that there is a right to reproduce.[43]

This conclusion is consistent with the fact that a right to reproduce is included in widely accepted manifestos of fundamental human rights. Consider the Universal Declaration of Human Rights, issued in 1948 by the General Assembly of the United Nations. Article 16, paragraph 1, states, "Men and women of full age, without any limitation due to race, nationality or religion, have the right to marry and to found a family."[44] The statement that there is a right "to found a family" implies a right to be free (at least within limits) from interference in procreating with one's marriage partner. A similar statement is found in article 12 of the European Convention on Human Rights: "Men and women of marriageable age have the right to marry and to found a family, according to the national laws governing the exercise of this right."[45] The above argument provides a justification for including a right to procreate in such manifestos.

Earlier it was noted that negative rights are prima facie claims. Accordingly, the above argument only yields the conclusion that there is a prima facie right to reproduce; it does not establish that the right is absolute. Yet, when we consider the importance of the reasons discussed above for valuing reproductive freedom, it is clear that the right should be regarded as very strong. If it can be overridden, doing so would require important reasons.

Interferences with the right to reproduce can vary in degree. At one extreme are interferences that are irreversible and highly intrusive of bodily integrity, such as hysterectomy. Clearly, this degree of interference, if performed against the wishes of a mentally competent person, would not be ethically justifiable in any situation we are likely to encounter. Other possible interferences are reversible or invade bodily integrity minimally or not at all. An example is the proposal that surrogate motherhood be forbidden. Proscribing gestational surrogacy arrangements would interfere with the right of some persons to reproduce, but it is a genuine issue as to whether such interference is ethically justifiable.[46] Another example involves disputes over frozen preembryos by divorcing couples. Any resolution of such disagreements is likely to interfere with the reproductive freedom of at least one party. Thus, it becomes a question of which interference is less objectionable. One of the important goals in each chapter of Part 2 will be to explore some possible limits to the right to reproduce. For example, some suggested limits of this right in the context of collaborative reproduction will be explored in Chapter 5, where I consider surrogacy and other nontraditional family arrangements. Similarly, limits associated with disputes over frozen preembryos will be discussed in Chapter 6. Having considered why freedom to procreate is important, we shall be better able in Part 2 to decide when the presumption in favor of freedom to procreate should be overridden.

Reasons why freedom not to procreate is important will be explored in the next chapter.

2

Constitutional and Women-Centered Perspectives

In 1957, Estelle Griswold became executive director of the Planned Parenthood League of Connecticut. She was described as a dynamic, vivacious woman strongly committed to opening Planned Parenthood clinics in that state.[1] However, her plans were obstructed by a Connecticut statute making it a crime to use any drug, medicinal article, or instrument for the purpose of preventing conception. Because of this law, the league's activities were limited to educational programs and a referral service to clinics in neighboring states. To challenge the statute, the Planned Parenthood League opened a clinic in New Haven on November 1, 1961, with Ms. Griswold as director and Dr. C. Lee Buxton, chairman of the Department of Obstetrics and Gynecology at the Yale University School of Medicine, as medical director. The services offered included providing contraceptives. Within ten days, Griswold and Buxton were arrested on charges of violating the statute as accessories by giving information, instruction, and advice to married persons for the purpose of contraception. The clinic was closed and Griswold and Buxton later were convicted and fined.

In forbidding contraceptive use, the Connecticut statute interfered with freedom not to procreate. In this chapter I want to explore why freedom not to procreate should be valued. In Chapter 1, I argued that freedom to procreate is valuable because of specific reasons that justify the desire to have children of one's own. Such reasons, however, do not explain why the desire *not* to have children should be respected. In exploring this topic, I shall distinguish between two senses of freedom not to procreate, along the lines of my previous distinction between two senses of freedom to procreate. Freedom not to procreate in the *strict* sense involves only the freedom to choose not to reproduce. In the *broad* sense, the term includes freedom to make additional choices associated with decisions not to procreate. For example, it includes freedom to obtain genetic information about oneself or one's fetus and to use that information in making a decision not to procreate. In this chapter, I shall focus on freedom not to procreate in the strict sense. Specifically, I want to explore why freedom not to beget and freedom not to gestate, both understood in the strict sense, are valuable to persons. The strategy is to try to understand why these fundamental senses of freedom not to procreate are important, and then to use this understanding in Part 2 to address some of the new issues involving freedom not to procreate in the broader sense.[2]

In exploring why freedom not to beget and freedom not to gestate should be valued, two sources are especially useful: constitutional law cases concerning procreation and feminist writings on reproductive ethics. A number of United States Supreme Court cases have dealt with the constitutional issues surrounding procreation. These cases and the legal literature concerning them provide insights into the ethical grounds of freedom not to beget and freedom not to gestate. Feminist writings place reproductive choices within a broader social context involving historical political and economic inequalities for women, and they draw our attention to special reasons why procreative freedom is important to women. These two sources bring to light different dimensions of the issue, and taken together they help us understand the importance of freedom not to procreate. Let us begin by considering the Supreme Court cases.

Griswold *and the Right to Privacy*

The seminal case dealing with freedom not to beget was *Griswold v. Connecticut,* decided by the U.S. Supreme Court in 1965.[3] In that case, Ms. Griswold and Dr. Buxton appealed their convictions for violating Connecticut's law against using contraceptives. Connecticut argued before the Court that the statute's purpose was to discourage extramarital relations. Banning contraceptives, it was claimed, helped prevent the indulgence by some in extramarital affairs. The Court found this argument unpersuasive, particularly in light of the admitted widespread availability in Connecticut of condoms for the prevention of disease, as opposed to prevention of conception. In its decision, the Court asserted for the first time that there is a constitutional right to privacy, a right which protects a married couple's decision to use contraceptives. The Court reversed the convictions and declared the Connecticut statute invalid, ruling that it unconstitutionally invaded the right to privacy of married persons. This decision marked the beginning of a line of Supreme Court cases which further elaborated upon the right to privacy and extended it to other areas involving procreation.

This was a remarkable decision and a source of controversy among constitutional scholars because nowhere in the Constitution is a right of marital privacy explicitly mentioned. Writing for the majority, Justice William O. Douglas argued that rights explicitly guaranteed in the Constitution and Bill of Rights have penumbras — associated rights that also are protected. For example, the First Amendment's freedoms of speech and press include not only freedom to utter and print, but also freedom to distribute, to receive, to read, to inquire, and to teach. Without these penumbral rights, the explicitly stated rights would be less secure. Similarly, it could be claimed that a right of marital privacy is protected by the Bill of Rights. Douglas argued that the Fourth Amendment explicitly guarantees the right of the people to be secure in their persons, houses, papers, and effects against unreasonable searches and seizures, and that this right creates a penumbral zone of privacy that includes the privacy of marital relationships. As Douglas put it: "Would we allow the police to search the sacred precincts of marital bedrooms for telltale signs of the use of contraceptives? The very idea is repulsive to the notions of privacy surrounding the marriage relationship."[4]

Moreover, the opinion asserted that the constitutional right to privacy is a *fundamental* right, which means that states must have especially strong justification for infringing it. When nonfundamental rights are infringed by statutes, the Supreme Court uses a less demanding test and regards a statute as constitutional provided it has some reasonable relation to the achievement of a proper state interest. For fundamental rights, however, the Court uses the test of strict scrutiny, which requires a compelling state interest to justify interference with the rights in question.[5]

In concurring opinions, Justices Arthur J. Goldberg, John M. Harlan, and Byron R. White stated that the right to privacy protects additional areas of family life that had been identified in previous Court decisions. In particular, the Justices referred to *Meyer v. Nebraska,* in which the Court had stated that the right to marry, establish a home, and bring up children is an important part of the liberty guaranteed by the Fourteenth Amendment. That case involved a Nebraska statute making it illegal to teach the German language to students below the eighth grade. In declaring the law unconstitutional, the Court in *Meyer* stated that it unreasonably encroached upon the freedom of parents to make decisions about the upbringing and education of their children.[6] In *Griswold,* the Justices asserted that this freedom is protected by the right to privacy.

Seven years after *Griswold,* the Court issued a decision extending the right to privacy to unmarried persons. *Eisenstadt v. Baird* dealt with the constitutionality of a Massachusetts law making it illegal to distribute contraceptives but containing an exception permitting physicians to prescribe contraceptives for married persons. The Court ruled that this law treated married and single persons differently and violated the Equal Protection Clause of the Fourteenth Amendment, which asserts that no state shall deny to any person within its jurisdiction the equal protection of the laws. The Supreme Court found the law unconstitutional and declared that all persons, married or single, have a right to use contraceptives. To quote the Court: "It is true that in Griswold the right of privacy in question inhered in the marital relationship. Yet the marital couple is not an independent entity with a mind and heart of its own, but an association of two individuals each with a separate intellectual and emotional makeup. If the right of privacy means anything, it is the right of the *individual,* married or single, to be free from unwarranted governmental intrusion into matters so fundamentally affecting a person as the decision whether to bear or beget a child."[7]

In additional cases, constitutional protections have been extended to other areas involving procreation. The right to privacy was held to protect the freedom to choose one's spouse in *Loving v. Virginia,* in which the Supreme Court struck down Virginia's ban on interracial marriages.[8] In *Stanley v. Illinois,* the Court overturned an Illinois law that authorized the removal of children from the custody of an unmarried natural father upon the death of the mother.[9] The Court held that an unwed natural father has a constitutionally protected interest in the custody of his children. And in *Roe v. Wade,* the Court dealt with the right not to gestate, establishing a constitutional right to abortion.

Roe v. Wade

Norma McCorvey, identified by the Court only as Jane Roe, was an unmarried pregnant woman who wanted to have an abortion. She was legally unable to do so because in Texas there was a criminal abortion statute prohibiting all abortions except those performed upon medical advice for the purpose of saving the mother's life. She initiated an action against Henry Wade, district attorney of Dallas County, in the U.S. District Court for the Northern District of Texas, seeking a declaratory judgment that the statute was unconstitutional and an injunction against its continued enforcement.

Appeals reached the U.S. Supreme Court, which issued a decision in 1973 written by Justice Harry Blackmun.[10]

The Court based its decision on the right to privacy established in *Griswold.* Justice Blackmun acknowledged the argument of *Griswold* that the right to privacy can be grounded on penumbras of the Bill of Rights, but chose instead to put forward an argument that had been stated in *Meyer v. Nebraska.* According to that argument, at least some rights that are not explicitly mentioned in the Constitution or Bill of Rights can be constitutionally grounded on the protection of liberty found in the Fourteenth Amendment's due process clause, which asserts that no state shall deprive any person of life, liberty, or property without due process of law.[11] Justice Blackmun asserted that the constitutional grounds of the right to privacy are thus found in the Fourteenth Amendment.

In *Roe,* the Court held that this right of privacy is broad enough to encompass a woman's decision whether to terminate her pregnancy.[12] The Court also recognized two state interests that must be balanced against a woman's right to privacy in the context of abortion. First, the state has an interest in upholding medical standards that protect the health of the pregnant woman. The Court ruled that, given current medical knowledge, this interest becomes compelling at approximately the end of the first trimester. Prior to this point in gestation, the mortality rate of abortions was less than that associated with pregnancy and childbirth. The Court ruled that after this point states can regulate abortions to the extent reasonably necessary to protect maternal health. Second, there is a state interest in protecting fetal life, which becomes compelling at viability. States that wish to protect fetal life after viability may forbid abortion during that period, except when it is necessary to preserve the life or health of the mother. The Texas statute was ruled unconstitutional because it did not distinguish between viable and previable fetuses and it permitted abortions only when necessary to save the mother's life.

A number of subsequent Supreme Court abortion cases have clarified and elaborated upon the ruling in *Roe.*[13] It is worth noting that part of the framework created in *Roe* and subsequent cases for balancing maternal and fetal interests was rejected by the Court in *Planned Parenthood of Southeastern Pennsylvania v. Casey.*[14] Prior to *Casey,* the Court had required strict scrutiny of all statutes that would place restrictions on abortion before viability. According to this approach, any statute creating an obstacle to a woman's right to abortion and not supported by compelling reasons would be considered unconstitutional. This had led to the Court's declaring unconstitutional such statutory requirements as twenty-four-hour waiting periods and provision of information that could be interpreted as having an anti-abortion bias. In *Casey,* the Court replaced strict scrutiny in this context with a new undue burden standard. According to this revised approach, statutes restricting abortion before viability are unconstitutional if they create a *substantial* obstacle to the woman's seeking an abortion.[15] Using this new standard, the Court in *Casey* upheld certain provisions of Pennsylvania's abortion law, including a twenty-four-hour waiting period and a requirement to make available to the woman information supporting a decision not to have an abortion.[16]

Following each decision since *Roe,* pro-choice and anti-abortion groups have debated the question of who won and lost. Despite the many decisions, including the introduction of the undue burden standard in *Casey,* the Court has never renounced the basic view stated in *Roe* that women have a constitutionally protected right to make decisions about abortion. The so-called right to privacy remains firm, but the Court's discussion of the theoretical basis of this right has been the source of yet another controversy.

Is Privacy the Basis of These Legal Procreative Rights?

As we have seen, a series of Supreme Court cases beginning with *Griswold* has based legal procreative rights on the concept of privacy. These rights have included rights not to procreate, such as a right to use contraceptives and a right to have abortions. However, the idea that the basis of these rights is the concept of privacy seems dubious. To see this, let us consider the meaning of privacy.

A number of commentators have attempted to define privacy, and there is a body of literature that critically assesses the strengths and weaknesses of various definitions.[17] An attempt to review this literature in detail would take us beyond the scope of the present discussion. My purpose is not to identify which version of the definition is best, but rather to utilize a central idea running through this literature. The central idea, stated in general terms, is this: Invasions of privacy involve the unjustifiable acquisition or dissemination of personal information about an individual. This idea is found in a number of definitions that have been put forward. For example, something close to it is implied by Elizabeth L. Beardsley's account, according to which violations of privacy consist of conduct by which one person Y acquires or discloses information about X which X does not wish to have known or disclosed.[18] Similarly, W. A. Parent defines the term as follows: Privacy is the condition of not having undocumented personal knowledge about oneself possessed by others. By undocumented, Parent means information that does not already belong to the public record.[19] The *right* to privacy, according to Parent, is the right not to have undocumented personal knowledge about ourselves unjustly or wrongly acquired by others.[20]

Given this central idea, let us consider whether the legal rights in question are based on privacy. Admittedly, privacy is relevant to the Connecticut law forbidding contraceptive use because enforcement of the law would require violations of privacy in the form of searches of marital bedrooms. Justice Douglas referred to this feature of the law and strongly opposed the idea of permitting such searches.[21] However, the legal right to decide whether to use contraceptives does not directly pertain to privacy. Rather, it involves a right to make certain decisions free of government interference. Moreover, these decisions do not directly involve disclosure of information about oneself; they involve procreative activity. Thus, the interest in question seems primarily to be autonomy, not privacy. A number of commentators, in fact, have argued that respect for autonomy provides the basis of the Court's decisions in *Griswold* and *Baird*.[22] Autonomy, or self-determination, refers to self-rule by an individual. It involves freedom from interference of others, as well as freedom from personal limitations such as lack of understanding that prevents informed choices.

When we consider *Roe,* it becomes even more apparent that the basis of these legal rights is autonomy rather than privacy. Like the earlier cases, *Roe* deals not with decisions that directly pertain to dissemination of information about oneself, but rather with procreative choices. However, privacy of the bedroom and home, which was a matter of grave concern in *Griswold,* is not even an issue in *Roe* because abortions are not performed in the home — at least, not legal ones. As noted above, Justice Blackmun explicitly stated in *Roe* that the right to privacy is based on the Fourteenth Amendment's protection of *liberty,* thereby rejecting Justice Douglas's penumbra argument.[23] However, in *Roe* and many subsequent cases the Court continued to refer to this liberty-based right as the right to privacy, thereby perpetuating confusion about the basis of its decisions in this area. In *Casey,* the court rested its justification of the right to abortion on liberty rather than privacy. Even here, however, the majority did not explicitly reject its previous use of the concept of privacy.[24]

My purpose is not to ascertain the best constitutional arguments for the legal rights in question; I refer the interested reader to the legal scholarship on that topic.[25] My concern is to identify ethical reasons supporting freedom not to beget and freedom not to gestate. The above discussion indicates that the ethical basis is autonomy rather than privacy. Also, I do not claim that privacy never would be violated by laws restricting these freedoms not to procreate, but that respect for autonomy provides the main ethical consideration against such laws.

Freedom not to beget and freedom not to gestate have a bearing on personal autonomy in several ways. First, these freedoms can be important for directing the course of one's life. The idea that some types of decisions typically are of central importance was expressed well by David A. J. Richards: "Certain choices in life are taken to bear fundamentally on the entire design of one's life, for these choices determine the basic decisions of work and love, which in turn order many of the subsidiary choices of human life. Obvious examples of such choices are matters of whether and where to be educated, choice of occupation and avocations, choice of whether and whom to love and befriend and on what terms, and the decision whether and to what extent children will be a life's concern."[26] Gestating and raising children is a large undertaking that competes with other important goals and projects in one's life by placing demands on time, energy, and resources. Thus, self-determination in making major life choices is promoted by freedom to decide whether to gestate and raise children (or, for those who have children, to gestate and raise *additional* children). Because begetting often leads to gestating and rearing, freedom not to beget is similarly important in making major life choices.

Second, the freedoms not to beget and not to gestate are important for *bodily* self-determination, a category of autonomy consisting of freedom to make decisions concerning what happens to one's body. Bodily self-determination is relevant, for example, to decisions concerning sterilization, birth control pills, and use of intrauterine devices. Although bodily self-determination applies to both men and women, it has special significance for women because they bear the burdens of gestation. As discussed in Chapter 1, pregnancy can be accompanied by somatic complaints such as fatigue, back-ache, heartburn, morning sickness, and other physical discomforts. Not only are these ailments disagreeable in themselves, but they can interfere with important activities. In addition, pregnancy alters body shape and poses risks to the woman's health. Bodily self-determination is implicated in decisions concerning abortion as well as contraception; the laws struck down in *Roe* and *Griswold* were morally objectionable in part because they interfered with the bodily self-determination of women.

It might be objected that freedom not to beget and freedom not to gestate are unnecessary for self-determination in making major life choices because children can be relinquished at birth for adoption. Thus, the burdens associated with child rearing could be avoided even if the state restricted the freedoms not to beget and not to gestate. In reply, relinquishing children admittedly provides an escape for some parents who wish to avoid child rearing. However, several considerations suggest that the availability of adoption does not necessarily free persons from the child-rearing tasks which follow from begetting and gestating. First, many people would find it psychologically difficult to relinquish a child at birth.[27] Parents often develop psychological attachments to their offspring during gestation. For some people, giving up a child would be emotionally traumatic, as illustrated by surrogate mothers who have refused to relinquish children they have gestated. Some who consider giving up a child might feel guilty, thinking that they would be shirking their responsibilities. Others might be distressed by the thought of having no voice or rights concerning the raising of children who are genetically their own. Thus, the fact that adoption is available does not mean that people are free from internal constraints which would prevent them from giving up their children. Second, there are social pressures which, for many people, would make it difficult to relinquish a child.[28] The parenthood prescription discussed in Chapter 1 would exert its influence, and many would feel pressure from friends and family not to give away their child. Thus, external forces as well as internal constraints reinforce our desires to raise our genetic offspring. It probably is a good thing that these pressures exist, because they reinforce the carrying out of our child-rearing responsibilities. Thus, the social conditioning which manifests itself as the parenthood prescription might have a positive side, insofar as it reinforces the nurturing of children. The objection in question overlooks these forces and assumes that giving up one's children is not difficult socially or psychologically. However, because giving up a child *is* difficult, freedom not to beget and freedom not to gestate are important for self-determination in making major life choices. This theme of self-determination is given an added dimension when we consider why freedom not to procreate is especially important to women, a topic to which we now turn.

Women-Centered Perspectives

For women to gain political, social, and economic equality in our society, it is essential that they have freedom to control their reproductive lives. Equality for women requires, among other things, greater integration of women into positions of authority and influence in all fields of endeavor. Because childbirth and child rearing require much time and energy, the more heavily one's life is devoted to these activities, the more difficult it is to pursue education and careers leading to positions of authority. Society generally has put little pressure on men to participate in child rearing, and women have shouldered most of the responsibilities in this area. For women as a group no longer to be held back, it is necessary that women be free to make their own decisions about when and whether to try to have children.

One of the first works to discuss the connection between reproductive roles and the subordination of women was Shulamith Firestone's *The Dialectic of Sex*. Firestone provided a historical analysis of the power difference between men and women. She argued that the domination of women by men is based on the different reproductive functions of males and females, arising from their biological differences with regard to procreation. As Firestone put it:

> The *biological family* — the basic reproductive unit of male/female/infant, in whatever form of social organization — is characterized by these fundamental — if not immutable facts: . . . That women throughout history before the advent of birth control were at the continual mercy of their biology — menstruation, menopause, and female ills, constant painful childbirth, wet-nursing and care of infants, all of which made them dependent on males (whether brother, father, husband, lover, or clan, government, community-at-large) for physical survival. . . . That the natural reproductive difference between the sexes led directly to the first division of labor at the origins of class, as well as furnishing the paradigm of caste (discrimination based on biological characteristics).[29]

Firestone envisioned an escape from these biological differences by means of the new reproductive technologies. She put forward the view that these technologies eventually would free women from pregnancy, childbirth, and child rearing. Conception and gestation entirely outside the womb would become possible. Moreover, the dependence of the child upon the mother would be replaced by alternative social arrangements for child rearing. These changes arising from reproductive technology would make possible the emergence of new and more equitable social roles for women. Firestone's work was highly influential in the 1970s. It was widely quoted by feminist writers, and it influenced some women to avoid childbearing in order to gain greater freedom for themselves. With passage of time, however, difficulties with Firestone's view have become apparent, and criticism by other feminists has become commonplace. Some point out that Firestone gives too much emphasis to seeking a technological fix. There is considerable skepticism among feminists that conception and complete gestation outside the uterus (ectogenesis), assuming it ever becomes possible, would automatically end male domination. It is pointed out that already there are a number of new reproductive technologies, such as in vitro fertilization and prenatal diagnosis. These technologies remain under the control of the male-dominated medical profession and, it is argued, have not moved women toward greater freedom. Contrary to Firestone, it is claimed that a more likely scenario for the future is that the new reproductive technologies will remain under male control. Not only is it asserted that Firestone's prediction will be inaccurate, but there is concern that these technologies actually will *increase* the social control of women by men.[30]

Other feminists oppose the part of Firestone's view which involves forsaking the experiences of pregnancy and childbirth. They argue that these experiences often are important and valuable to women. They seek a way of liberating women that does not require giving up these experiences. Adrienne Rich, for example, distinguishes between the *experience* of motherhood, which may be desirable for many women, and the *institution* of motherhood — the social practices surrounding motherhood by which men have exploited women. She and others argue that to liberate women it is not necessary to eliminate pregnancy and childbirth. Rather, the oppressive aspects of the institution of motherhood must be removed.[31] As one feminist proclamation puts it, "We do not need to transform our biology, we need to transform patriarchal, social, political, and economic conditions."[32]

As these disagreements suggest, there is no such thing as *the* feminist view. Rather, there are a variety of views, as further illustrated by considering some main types of feminism. Alison M. Jaggar and Paula Rothenberg Struhl distinguish four feminist frameworks and contrast them with a nonfeminist viewpoint which they refer to as conservatism.[33] Conservatism attempts to justify women's position in contemporary society by arguing that it is based on some type of biological imperative. *Liberal feminism* recognizes that women historically have been unfairly treated, and it emphasizes that the liberation of women requires that they have equal opportunities for education and professional advancement. *Marxist feminists* hold that the main source of women's oppression is class division and the exploitation of the majority by those who own the means of production. Hence, they argue that liberation for women would be achieved by a revolution that abolishes private property and establishes public ownership of the means of production. *Radical feminists* disagree. They believe that women can be oppressed in any type of economic system. They assert that women's oppression is a result of the biological difference between men and women in regard to childbearing ability. Therefore, the liberation of women requires either a freedom from our biology through new reproductive technologies (Firestone) or abolition of the oppressive institution of motherhood (Rich). Finally, *social feminists* accept a Marxist connection between class society and sexism but deny that sexism is the less fundamental. On this view, the liberation of women requires the elimination both of class society and of the oppressive institution of childbearing and rearing.[34]

In addition to disagreements concerning theoretical underpinnings, there are differing views concerning specific issues. Some feminists see the new reproductive technologies as a severe threat and fear that these techniques will be used to increase the subjugation of women. They assert that women already have been exploited in the development of these technologies, and they bolster this view by emphasizing the risks to women in techniques such as in vitro fertilization. Some view the new reproductive technologies as a declaration of war against women by the male-dominated medical profession. They see themselves as activists and advocate a complete rejection of all new reproductive technologies and research concerning them.[35] Other feminists criticize these views on several grounds. First, these activists sometimes overstate the risks or fail to document their claims about risks. Second, the activists tend to consider only the risks, overlooking the benefits to women from reproductive technology. Their critics point out, for example, that artificial insemination by donor has provided a beneficial means to alternative family arrangements for some single and lesbian women; that in vitro fertilization has brought children into the lives of some infertile women; that abortion has been instrumental in preserving health and improving the lives of women; and that contraception has given women greater freedom to avoid pregnancy. A number of feminists argue that an outright rejection of all reproductive technologies would be wrong, and that all women, including the poor, should have access to them.[36]

Another issue about which feminists are divided is surrogate motherhood. The activists tend to see surrogacy as dehumanizing to the surrogate, the child, and women and children generally. They believe that surrogacy exploits the surrogate mother and that surrogacy for money should be prohibited.[37] By contrast, some feminists defend surrogacy, arguing that forbidding it would interfere with the reproductive autonomy of women. They argue that a contractual agreement whereby the surrogate mother relinquishes custody of the child to the infertile couple should be legally enforceable. To make such agreements unenforceable, it is claimed, would be paternalistic and would reinforce the old argument used against women that they are unable to make decisions.[38]

Although there is diversity of views, it is important to take note of common themes that run through the feminist literature on reproductive ethics. Several authors have attempted to identify these main ideas, and I draw upon their work in order to point out the following feminist themes.[39]

1. A feminist perspective is founded upon an awareness that women have been and are the victims of oppression under a system of male dominance, the term *oppression* referring to unjustified limitations and barriers.
2. A feminist perspective seeks the removal of the oppression of women and the bringing about of sexual equality.
3. With regard to reproduction in particular, women should not be exploited. Women should have control over their bodies, gametes, and conceptuses. Women should have not only freedom to procreate but also the freedoms not to beget and not to gestate. Moreover, modern obstetrics is characterized by a loss of control by women associated with the increasing medicalization of pregnancy and childbirth. Feminists assert that this medicaliza-

tion has gone too far, and that women should gain greater control over pregnancy and childbirth.

4. In formulating policies concerning reproductive ethical issues, greater attention must be given to the input of women concerning their needs, interests, and perspectives. More consideration must be given to the question of how new reproductive technologies and policies will affect women. In the development of these policies, women must play a prominent role.

These themes, which are neither exhaustive nor mutually exclusive, generally have received little attention in the literature of mainstream medical ethics. That literature largely has been silent about male dominance in medicine. Few authors writing on medical ethics have been critical of practices that contribute to the oppression of women. Mainstream medical ethics must begin to give adequate consideration to these feminist concerns.

I have argued that freedom not to beget and freedom not to gestate are important for the self-determination of men and women because bearing and raising children is a large task, the undertaking of which can compete with other important life tasks by placing demands on time and resources. For women, these freedoms are particularly important because they are essential for social change toward equality for women. In addition, bodily self-determination is especially significant for women because they are the ones whose bodies support the developing fetus during gestation. In Chapter 1, I argued that freedom to procreate can be important to one's self-identity and self-fulfillment. Similarly, the freedoms not to beget and not to gestate are significant for self-identity and self-fulfillment because they involve major life decisions. For women in particular, these freedoms are crucial to self-identity and self-fulfillment as women seek new, more equitable, social roles for themselves. Both freedom to procreate and freedom not to procreate are valuable, ultimately, because of their importance for the self-determination of persons.

The discussion of rights in Chapter 1 can be applied to the question of whether there is a right not to beget and a right not to gestate. I argued that persons have a moral right to be free from any interference that would constitute treating them as mere means and not as ends in themselves. Several considerations support the view that interfering with freedom not to beget and freedom not to gestate constitutes a failure to treat persons as ends in themselves. First, depriving persons of the ability to make the important decision not to have a child would be an interference with self-determination and self-fulfillment. To interfere with persons' lives in this major way would be a failure to provide the full respect due to them. Second, to interfere with the ability of women to gain equality by denying them the freedoms not to beget and not to gestate would be a failure to treat them as ends in themselves. These considerations support the view that there are prima facie rights not to beget and not to gestate.

In the first two chapters we have considered why procreative freedom is worthy of protection. We have identified important reasons why there should be a presumption in favor of freedom to procreate and the freedoms not to beget and not to gestate. Another matter we need to consider is the moral status of offspring during and after gestation, a topic that I shall take up in the next chapter.

3

The Moral Standing of Embryos, Fetuses, and Infants

Few topics in medical ethics have received as much attention as the moral status of the fetus. In fact, some authors believe that too much has been written about this topic and not enough about the interests of pregnant women.[1] Nevertheless, reproductive ethics cannot be discussed adequately without considering the moral standing of the fetus. In this chapter, I present and defend a view on the moral status of embryos and fetuses.

Some believe that we can sidestep the issue of the fetus's moral status. M. E. Winston, for example, suggests that our obligations to fetuses can be ascertained by looking instead at the responsibilities of procreators toward their offspring.[2] Winston argues that whenever persons, through their own free action, are directly and foreseeably causally responsible for the creation of offspring, they have parental responsibilities toward those offspring. These responsibilities include an obligation to protect the offspring from harm and to exercise reasonable care to promote the offspring's development toward maturity. This implies, according to Winston, that pregnant women have a prima facie duty not to abort a conceptus or fetus unless the act leading to conception was not voluntary, the woman was mentally incompetent, or there was contraceptive failure. Abortion outside of such exceptional circumstances would constitute a prima facie violation of parental responsibility and hence be wrong.

However, Winston's attempt to avoid dealing with the moral standing of embryos and fetuses does not succeed. Because the parental obligations he claims exist are prima facie, the question arises concerning what ethical considerations override them. Many who hold a pro-choice view concerning abortion argue that embryos have a relatively low moral status and that therefore almost any reason justifies a woman's decision to abandon her obligations and abort the pregnancy during the embryonic period. Thus, deciding whether it is justifiable to abandon such obligations requires addressing the question of the embryo's moral status. Similar questions about moral standing arise in regard to overriding parental obligations during other stages of pregnancy, as well.

Arguments concerning the moral status of embryos and fetuses can be religious or secular; mine are the latter. Some groundwork must be laid before I state the specifics of my view, but in general terms it holds that moral status increases as the fetus develops during pregnancy. Different versions of this view are possible, but I do not embrace them all. For example, some versions are referred to as gradualist, based on the fact that fetal development is gradual and continuous. Norman Gillespie puts forward such a view and defends it by means of the following principle: if x units of some property Q justify that one have x units of some right or duty E, then y units of Q justify that one have y units of E.[3] Gillespie does not attempt to identify the property Q that supposedly increases during pregnancy, but he seems to believe that there is such a property and that as it increases the right to life of the fetus increases proportionately. I do not apply the term *gradualist* to my view, nor do I utilize Gillespie's principle of proportionality, because they imply that fetal moral standing increases linearly with development — that is, in direct proportion to the degree of development. To say that moral standing increases linearly implies distinctions that seem too fine. It implies, for example, that a sixteen-cell preembryo has greater moral standing than a four-cell preembryo — perhaps only slightly greater, but nevertheless greater. It implies that with each minor increase in development of fetal organs there is a corresponding increase in the fetus's moral standing. However, it is not at all clear that such minor differences should count, morally. The gradualist view also implies that there are no significant milestones along the course of fetal development that have special moral significance. The view that I shall defend does not have these implications. Although I draw upon the work of others, I shall attempt to put forward an original way of thinking about progressively increasing moral standing.

The view that fetal moral status increases during pregnancy is widely held, and deservedly so, given that it has a certain intuitive plausibility. In particular, an attractive feature of this view is its agreement with widely held moral intuitions concerning embryos, fetuses, and infants, such as the following: use of intrauterine devices seems morally unobjectionable, even though this birth control method causes the nonimplantation and death of the preembryo; abortion early in gestation is less problematic ethically than late abortion; in cases where continuing gestation threatens the pregnant woman's life, her life takes priority over the fetus's life; fetuses near term have a moral standing that is close to, if not the same as, that of infants; and infanticide generally is wrong. Despite the attractiveness of the view that moral standing increases as gestation proceeds, little attention has been given to articulating it clearly and justifying it.

Views on When Moral Standing Begins

To lay the groundwork referred to above, it is necessary to review briefly some of the views that have been put forward concerning when moral standing begins. An approach taken by a number of authors is to argue that a right to life is acquired when some special characteristic is obtained. It will be helpful to consider the main characteristics that have been proposed, in order to understand not only their shortcomings but the insights they provide. Although I shall argue that none of the views in question are correct, they have a bearing on the view I shall defend.

SELF-CONSCIOUSNESS

A prominent view is that individuals acquire a right to life upon becoming self-conscious. The best-known advocate is Michael Tooley, who states, "An organism possesses a serious right to life only if it possesses the concept of a self as a continuing subject of experiences and other mental states, and believes that it is itself such a continuing entity."[4] Based on this view, Tooley argues that fetuses lack a right to life and that abortion is morally permissible.

However, a serious difficulty with this view is its implications for infants. Because infants lack self-consciousness they also fail to have a serious right to life, according to Tooley's account. This conclusion is at odds with our moral intuitions that killing infants is wrong. The view that infants have serious moral interests that should be protected is widely held. It has been a prominent view, for example, in discussions of the Baby Doe issue, where it has been the basis of position statements by the President's Commission for the Study of Ethical Problems in Medicine and the Hastings Center Research Project on the Care of Imperiled Newborns.[5] Among the general public, such intuitions seem widespread, as reflected in the fact that the law regards newborns as legal persons.

When a philosophical theory — in particular, the theory that infants lack a right to life because they lack self-consciousness — conflicts with strongly held intuitions, we should ask whether the theory is compelling enough to outweigh those intuitions.[6] In addressing this question, we should consider whether there is a basis other than self-consciousness upon which our intuitions about infants can be grounded. If these intuitions can be satisfactorily defended by ethical arguments, that defense will support the rejection of Tooley's view. I shall argue below that these intuitions can be defended.

Although Tooley's view seems mistaken in making self-consciousness a necessary condition for a right to life, it conveys the important point that self-consciousness is *sufficient* for a right to life. Perhaps the most straightforward way to defend this claim is to consider a paradigm of self-conscious individuals, namely, normal adult human beings. We self-conscious adult humans are ends in ourselves because of the things we can do, things that go along with being self-conscious agents: we can formulate goals and preferences based on rational deliberation and values we select; we have the ability to choose plans based on our values and beliefs, including broad plans concerning the conduct of our lives; and we are capable of rationally taking steps to pursue our plans and advance the values we deem important. We are examples of self-legislating rational beings in the Kantian sense, beings who should be treated with full moral respect. The same moral standing would be possessed, of course, by any extraterrestrial or other nonhuman self-conscious individuals, if any exist. Self-conscious individuals have full moral standing because they have these intrinsic qualities.

POTENTIAL FOR SELF-CONSCIOUSNESS

A number of authors have argued that the *potential* for self-consciousness gives individuals full moral standing, including a right to life. Philip E. Devine, for example, states the potentiality principle as follows: "According to this principle, there is a property, self-consciousness or the use of speech for instance, such that (i) it is possessed by adult humans, (ii) it endows any organism possessing it with a serious right to life, and (iii) it is such that any organism potentially possessing it has a serious right to life even now — where an organism possesses a property potentially if it will come to have that property under normal conditions for development."[7]

One reply to the potentiality argument claims that it is based on a logical mistake. As H. Tristram Engelhardt, Jr., puts it, "If X is a potential Y, it follows that X is not a Y. If fetuses are potential persons, it follows clearly that fetuses are not persons. As a consequence, X does not have the actual rights of Y, but only potentially has the rights of Y."[8] However, as Bonnie Steinbock points out, the potentiality argument need not be based on this logical mistake.[9] Those who put forward the potentiality argument can be understood as making a normative claim, to the effect that individuals having the potential to become self-conscious *ought* to have the same moral status as those who already are self-conscious.

Another response to the potentiality argument is that it leads to conclusions about sperm and ova that are at odds with our intuitions. Helga Kuhse and Peter Singer put forward this view, beginning with the premise that sperm and ova do not have a right to life.[10] Kuhse and Singer ask us to consider semen and an ovum immediately after they have been combined in a petri dish. In the normal course of events, if things go well, a sperm will penetrate the egg and fertilize it. Kuhse and Singer claim that the set of entities consisting of the semen and ovum have the potential to develop into a self-conscious individual, just as a fertilized ovum (zygote) does. If the ovum and sperm have this potential and it is not wrong to destroy them, then the zygote's potential does not make it wrong for it to be destroyed.

However, this argument based on our moral intuitions concerning sperm and ova does not refute all forms of the potentiality argument. Two senses of potentiality are distinguished by Stephen Buckle: potential *to become* and potential *to produce*.[11] The former sense assumes the existence of an entity that maintains its identity over time, but the latter sense does not make this assumption. Buckle describes the distinction as follows:

> The power to become is the power possessed by an entity to undergo changes which are changes to itself, that is, to undergo growth or, better still, development. The potential to become can thus be called developmental potential. The process of actualizing the potential to become preserves some form of individual identity. It is for this reason that the potential to become is peculiarly appropriate to arguments which are concerned to establish the importance of respecting the capacities of a specific individual. The potential to produce differs in precisely this respect — it does not require that any form of identity be preserved. . . . A mixture of gases, if it includes hydrogen and oxygen, has the potential to produce water.[12]

As Buckle points out, these two senses reflect two different reasons why one might think potentiality is morally important. The first is deontological and holds that an existing being should be respected because it has the potential to develop into a being that deserves respect in its own right. On this view, the existing being should be respected because it is the same being as the later being into which it develops, and therefore it is considered to have moral standing. The second type of reason is consequentialist and gives moral significance to whatever has the potential to produce good or bad outcomes. Although the potential to produce a self-conscious entity has moral significance, it is not the type of significance that attaches to respect for individuals, but rather is the type of significance that figures in calculations of best outcomes. That significance reflects the value of possible future states of affairs and does not entail, for example, that an embryo has a right to life.[13]

Although the sperm and ovum, as well as the zygote, have the potential *to produce* a self-conscious individual, they lack the potential *to become* a self-conscious individual. The reason is that the zygote is not the same individual as the embryo proper. As Buckle points out, as cell division proceeds following fertilization, cells begin to differentiate in order to carry out a range of functions. Some cells or their descendants form the placenta, while others become yolk sac, others amnion, and so forth. It is only in a subset of cells, the embryonic plate, that the so-called primitive streak appears, marking the beginning of the embryo itself. The embryo is distinct from the other life-support structures such as the placenta, amnion, and chorion. If the zygote can be said to be identical to some entity, it would seem to be the entity consisting of the entire collection of cells derived from it. However, this entity is not the same as the embryo proper, which is the part that develops into a self-conscious individual.[14]

Thus, Kuhse and Singer's argument that the zygote lacks a right to life does not refute all forms of the potentiality argument. It only refutes a version that employs the concept of potential to produce, since that is the only potential for self-consciousness that a zygote has. Kuhse and Singer's argument has value, however, because it helps us see clearly that potential to produce self-consciousness is not grounds for a right to life.

Advocates of the potentiality argument can respond to Kuhse and Singer by focusing on the embryo proper and claiming that it has the potential to become a self-conscious individual. They would then argue that the embryo proper ought to have the same moral status as a self-conscious individual because of this potential. We need to consider, therefore, how to respond to this version of the potentiality argument.

I suggest a two-pronged attack. First, it is not enough simply to claim that the potential to become an individual with self-consciousness constitutes grounds for moral standing; an argument is needed. However, it seems that no satisfactory argument has been given. Let us consider, for example, the arguments put forward by Devine, of which there seem to be two. One argument begins with the moral intuition that infants should be protected by the rule against homicide. He points out that support for the potentiality principle derives from the fact that it can account for this moral intuition; although infants do not possess self-consciousness, they have the potential to acquire it.[15] In reply, there might be alternative ways to justify the protection of infants against homicide. If there is an alternative justification, then one need not accept the potentiality principle. In what follows, I shall argue that there is another justification.

Devine's second argument is stated as follows: "The basis of the potentiality principle is quite simple; what makes the difference between human beings and other life is the capacity human beings enjoy for a specially rich kind of life. The life already enjoyed by a human being cannot be taken away from him, only the prospect of such life in the future. But this prospect is possessed as much by an infant or fetus as by a full-grown adult."[16] In reply, individuals possessing self-consciousness and individuals possessing the potential to become self-conscious are not deprived of the same thing when they are killed. Individuals possessing self-consciousness are deprived of the *continuation* of ongoing plans and projects. They typically are deprived of the continuation of highly developed social relationships with family, friends, and other individuals. Killing them involves negating the ends that already have been chosen by self-legislating rational beings. Killing an individual who has never possessed self-consciousness but has the potential for it does not involve any of these things. Therefore, it is a mistake to say that what is taken away from the two types of individuals is the same. Thus, Devine's second argument is unsuccessful.

The second prong is to point out that the argument in question leads to conclusions at odds with our moral intuitions. An example similar to one suggested by Leonard Glantz will illustrate the point nicely.[17] Let us suppose that technological advances make it possible to keep an embryo proper alive in vitro, at least for a short period of time. Let us suppose, also, that it becomes technically feasible to transfer such an embryo to a woman's uterus, so that it has the potential to become a self-conscious individual. Now, suppose that a fire breaks out in the laboratory where one of these embryos is being kept alive. You enter the laboratory and see a ten-year-old child lying on the floor, suffering from the smoke and heat. You face a choice: either to carry out the embryo with the life-support equipment to which it is attached or to carry out the child. Clearly, the morally correct choice is to rescue the child. This example shows that the embryo's potential to become a self-conscious individual does not give it full moral standing.

Nevertheless, an important insight provided by the argument from potential is that the potential to produce and the potential to become a self-conscious individual are morally relevant characteristics, in part because they enter into consequentialist considerations about future outcomes. Another conclusion of the above discussion is that the preembryo, which is the product of gametic union from fertilization until the formation of the primitive streak,[18] does not have the potential *to become* a self-conscious individual because it is not identical to the embryo proper.

SENTIENCE

Others have argued that fetuses acquire a right to life upon becoming sentient. I shall use the term *sentience* to mean the capacity for feeling or perceiving. A creature that is capable of experiencing any of the five senses or pain or sensations of pleasure is sentient. Synonyms for sentience include *awareness* and *consciousness*. Sentience is not the same as self-consciousness, which involves reflection on oneself and one's sensations. L. W. Sumner has defended sentience as the basis of the right to life.[19] According to Sumner, to have moral standing is to have a right to life, but different types of creatures have different degrees of moral standing and hence a right to life with different strength. Moreover, to have sentience is to have moral standing, and the difference in moral standing between different types of creatures is due to the fact that they have different degrees of sentience. As Sumner puts it:

> Within any given mode, such as the perception of pain, one creature may be more or less sensitive than another. But there is a further sense in which more developed (more rational) creatures possess a higher degree of sentience. The expansion of consciousness and of intelligence opens up new ways of experiencing the world, and therefore new ways of being affected by the world. More rational beings are capable of finding either fulfillment or frustration in activities and states of affairs to which less developed creatures are, both cognitively and affectively, blind. It is in this sense of a broader and deeper sensibility that a higher being is capable of a richer, fuller, and more varied existence. The fact that sentience admits of degrees . . . enables us to employ it . . . as a comparison criterion of moral standing. The animal kingdom presents us with a hierarchy of sentience. Nonsentient beings have no moral standing; among sentient beings the more developed have greater standing than the less developed.[20]

Sumner states that, based on current information, fetuses seem to acquire sentience at some time during the second trimester. He concludes that fetuses late in the second trimester and in the third trimester have a right to life. Abortion during that stage of pregnancy is morally justifiable, according to Sumner, only for weighty reasons such as a serious threat to the woman's life or health or a risk of serious fetal deformity.[21]

However, there is a problem with this attempt to ground the fetus's moral standing on sentience. Sumner assigns to late-second-trimester fetuses a right to life that is close in strength to that of normal adult humans. This implies that a right to life of similar strength should be assigned to nonhuman animals that have a degree of sentience comparable to that of late-second-trimester human fetuses. But the human fetus is only beginning to develop sentience at that point, and surely adult members of many nonhuman animal species have at least as great a degree of sentience. Sumner's view, therefore, seems to commit him to the position that, for example, adult cattle, sheep, and cats should have a right to life that is very close to that of normal adult humans. Admittedly, there are some people who hold this view, but it is highly question-able and certainly at odds with the moral intuitions of many. We need a better account of the moral standing of human fetuses, one that does not focus exclusively on sentience and that accounts for our moral intuitions about fetuses without committing us to questionable views concerning the moral standing of nonhuman animals.

Nevertheless, the sentience criterion provides important insights. As Joel Feinberg has convincingly argued, only sentient creatures are capable of hav-ing moral interests. In his words, "an interest, however the concept is finally to be analyzed, presupposes at least rudimentary cognitive equipment. Interests are compounded out of *desires* and *aims,* both of which presuppose something like *belief,* or cognitive awareness."[22] Thus, one difference between sentient and nonsentient fetuses is that the former have moral interests but the latter do not. Having interests cannot be equated with having a right to life, but it is relevant to the fetus's moral standing, as we shall see.

VIABILITY

Viability was put forward as a significant dividing line in the 1973 U.S. Supreme Court *Roe v. Wade* decision. According to the majority opinion written by Justice Blackmun, a fetus becomes viable when it is potentially able to live outside the mother's womb, albeit with artificial aid.[23] Moreover, the Court declared that viability is the point at which the state's interest in poten-tial life becomes compelling enough to override the pregnant woman's right to self-determination, allowing states to forbid abortion following viability ex-cept when it is necessary to protect the life or health of the mother. Although this is a legal ruling, it seems to be based on the idea that viability is morally significant.

The view that viability is a criterion of moral standing faces several diffi-culties. First, as Norman Fost and his colleagues point out, the logic of the viability criterion is puzzling. As they put it, "Why should a fetus's capacity to live independently be a reason to forbid the mother from forcing it to live independently?"[24] In considering the previable fetus, Devine makes a similar point: "There is no reason to suppose that the fact that a given creature cannot live outside a given environment provides a reason why depriving it of that environment should be morally acceptable."[25]

Another objection, stated by Roger Wertheimer, is that future technological advances conceivably could place viability much earlier in pregnancy.[26] To use a rather futuristic example, suppose that an embryo could be kept alive and its development supported extracorporally until term. The viability criterion would then require us to say that embryos have the same moral standing as normal adult human beings, an implausible conclusion. Alan Zaitchik has attempted to respond to this objection.[27] According to Zaitchik, those who advocate the viability criterion do not infer the personhood of the viable fetus from a general thesis concerning necessary and sufficient conditions for personhood. Rather, they react by seeing the viable fetus as a person. What they are reacting to is a complex set of possible interactions between ourselves and the fetus, for we can easily imagine it already outside its mother's body and being maintained by artificial support. We can imagine handling, feeding, and caring for it as a newborn. This set of interactions might be absent or at least very different if we were dealing with a viable embryo being maintained extracorporally. Therefore, says Zaitchik, those who advocate the viability criterion would not be committed to recognizing the viable embryo as a person. However, Zaitchik's argument amounts to a concession that viability is not a criterion of moral standing. According to his argument, it is not viability itself that matters, but viability combined with a relatively advanced stage of fetal development.[28]

Laurence B. McCullough and Frank A. Chervenak have argued that fetuses acquire moral status when they become viable. This argument is part of their attempt to base the moral status of fetuses on the concept of being a patient.[29] They begin with the premise that physicians owe beneficence-based obligations to their patients. Once it is ascertained that a particular fetus should be regarded as a patient, according to McCullough and Chervenak, something significant is known about that fetus's moral status — namely, that its physician owes beneficence-based obligations to it. They hold that the physician's obligations to the fetal patient are seemingly on a par with the physician's obligations to the pregnant woman.[30]

McCullough and Chervenak claim that an individual becomes a patient when two conditions are satisfied: when the individual is (1) presented to a physician (2) for the purpose of applying clinical interventions that are reliably expected to protect and promote the interests of that individual.[31] On their view, there are two ways in which a fetus can satisfy these conditions. First, a previable fetus can satisfy them if the pregnant woman makes an autonomous decision to confer the status of being a patient on her fetus. The pregnant woman is free to confer or withhold this status, and once she confers it, she is free to withdraw it, as long as the fetus is previable. The first condition for patienthood is satisfied when the pregnant woman presents herself and the fetus to the physician. To show that the second condition can be satisfied for the fetus, McCullough and Chervenak argue that the previable fetus can have interests. They claim that when the pregnant woman has made a *settled* decision to confer the status of being a patient upon her previable fetus, there is a *link* between the fetus and the future individual it will become, who at some point will possess self-consciousness, which is necessary and sufficient for independent moral status. The link, specifically, is that such fetuses are reliably expected to achieve independent moral status.[32] When achieving independent moral status is reliably expected, they claim, the fetus has a present interest in achieving that status.

The second way that a fetus can become a patient, according to McCullough and Chervenak, is by becoming viable. They hold that viability is relevant because it also establishes a link between the fetus and the future individual who will have independent moral status. Again, the link is that the fetus is reliably expected to achieve independent moral status, and they claim that the fetus has a present interest in achieving that status. As they put it, the viable fetus has interests, derived from the biologic-technologic capacity to later achieve independent moral status, that can reliably be expected to be protected and promoted by obstetric interventions.[33] Thus, the second condition for patienthood is fulfilled. Moreover, they claim that the first condition is fulfilled not only when the pregnant woman presents herself and the fetus to the physician, but whenever the pregnant woman is reasonably thought to be *obligated* to present the viable fetus to the physician for the purpose of applying interventions.

There are several serious difficulties with this view put forward by McCullough and Chervenak. Let us begin with their discussion of previable fetuses. Because some, if not all, previable fetuses are presentient, their view entails that presentient fetuses can have interests. However, many readers will regard this as implausible, particularly those who accept Feinberg's analysis, according to which individuals must be sentient to have interests. McCullough and Chervenak do not acknowledge this problem, and they make no attempt to reconcile their view with Feinberg's. Because they do not address this obvious objection, their argument that previable fetuses can have moral status is unsuccessful.

A second problem is that McCullough and Chervenak fail to consider thoroughly the question concerning *to whom* the physician owes an obligation to act beneficently toward the previable fetus. When a pregnant woman with a previable fetus presents herself to an obstetrician and a physician-patient relationship is established, it is reasonable to hold that the physician undertakes an obligation to the woman to act beneficently toward her fetus. Moreover, one can seemingly account for the fetus's role as patient in terms of such an obligation. If the obligation is owed to the woman and not to the fetus, then one need not conclude that the fetus has moral status. McCullough and Chervenak assume that an obligation is owed to the previable fetus, and they do not consider the possibility that the fetus could occupy the role of patient without the physician's obligation being owed directly to it. Their failure to consider this possibility represents another way in which they do not satisfactorily defend their view.

Their view has additional implications that seem implausible. For one thing, it implies that a fetus at *any point in gestation, no matter how early,* can have significant moral status provided the woman has made a settled decision to continue the pregnancy and presents herself to an obstetrician for care that is reliably expected to promote the health of the fetus. This implies that some fetuses early in gestation can have the same degree of moral status as fetuses late in gestation. Moreover, their view implies that some previable fetuses at a given gestational age that have been presented to an obstetrician have moral status, while other fetuses at the same gestational age lack moral status simply because they have not been presented to an obstetrician.

There also is a difficulty with their argument that viability gives rise to moral status. It is worth noting that when a pregnant woman presents her viable fetus to an obstetrician for care, it is not viability alone that gives rise to moral status, according to McCullough and Chervenak. Rather, it is viability plus the fact that the woman has presented the fetus to the obstetrician.[34] However, when the woman has an *obligation* to present the fetus for care, her actually presenting it is *not* a necessary condition for the fetus's moral status, on their view. In this situation, their view implies that the fact of viability by itself is sufficient to mount an argument for the fetus's moral status. However, there is a problem with the claim that the pregnant woman has an obligation to present the fetus for health care. Where does this obligation come from? It cannot be based on the fetus's moral status as a patient, because that status comes into being only if it has been established that the woman has an obligation to present the viable fetus for care (assuming that she does not actually present it). If the fetus is not a patient, then it has no moral status, according to McCullough and Chervenak, because it lacks the self-consciousness necessary for independent moral status. Thus, McCullough and Chervenak beg the question when they assert that a viable fetus that has not been presented for care has moral status because the woman has an obligation to present it for care. Their attempt to show that viability by itself can provide the basis of a valid argument for moral status fails.

The above considerations support the view that viability by itself is not a satisfactory criterion of moral standing. Nevertheless, the discussion suggests several ways in which a fetus's attaining viability, currently at the gestational age of approximately twenty-two to twenty-four weeks, is *morally relevant*. First, viability is an identifiable stage at which the fetus is recognized as being relatively advanced in development. Second, with viability the fetus's social role increases to some extent, particularly its role as a patient. This arises because of several contingent facts: because abortion on demand is not a legal option, pregnant women with viable fetuses are normally expected eventually to give birth to live infants; and with the onset of viability, there is an increase in the number of possible medical interventions for the sake of the fetus, including early delivery. These facts help generate a reasonable attitude on the part of physicians that the viable fetus is a patient. Thus, as it becomes viable, its social role as a patient becomes somewhat more secure.

Conferred Moral Status

We have seen that none of the above views provides an adequate account of moral standing. In looking for an alternative account, it will be helpful to make two distinctions. First, we need to distinguish between two senses of the term *personhood*. The first sense is normative and refers to a moral status that we might call full moral standing. It involves having a substantial set of rights, including but not limited to a strong right to life. The second sense is descriptive and refers to the possession of self-consciousness, which typically is accompanied by other attributes, including use of language, capacity for rational thought and action, ability to profess values, and moral agency. Those who are self-conscious are persons in both senses of the term. Steinbock has suggested the terms *normative* and *descriptive* personhood, respectively, to refer to these two senses, and I shall use these terms.[35]

The second distinction is between *intrinsic* and *conferred* moral standing. In the above discussion of the self-consciousness criterion, I argued that self-conscious individuals have full moral standing because of their inherent characteristics. One might say that self-conscious individuals have intrinsic moral standing because of the characteristics they possess. By contrast, it is conceivable that some individuals should be regarded as having moral status not because they have intrinsic moral standing but because it is justifiable to confer moral status upon them.[36]

If embryos, fetuses, and infants have moral standing, it cannot be on the basis of their inherent characteristics alone, for they lack the characteristics needed for intrinsic moral standing; they are not persons in the descriptive sense. It is necessary, therefore, to consider whether it is justifiable to confer some degree of moral standing upon them. Should fetuses and infants be regarded as persons in the normative sense, even though they are not persons in the descriptive sense?

Let us consider how conferred moral standing for individuals who are not descriptive persons can be justified. I suggest that one might take two main approaches. First, several authors have argued that conferring moral standing on infants and at least some fetuses might be justified by the *consequences* of doing so. S. I. Benn, for example, suggests that one reason for treating infants with consideration and tenderness is the good consequences this might have for the persons they grow up to become. Persons who are deprived of love and tender care as infants might become emotionally stunted or impaired. As Benn puts it: ". . . it is for the sake of those that will grow into persons that we take care of all babies now. For not to do so for some—those that we regard as expendable or dispensable [sic]—might well lead us into a callous unconcern for others too."[37] Benn goes on to say that if such a case can be made for infants, it might also be made for fetuses, at least those at a stage of maturity at which "we can reasonably associate the way we treat them with the way we treat babies—at a stage, that is, at which we think of them, vividly enough, as a baby in the womb."[38]

In commenting on Benn's idea, Feinberg voices his agreement and adds that if infants are not treated with tenderness, then "when they are adults, others will suffer for it too, at their hands. Spontaneous warmth and sympathy toward babies then clearly has a great deal of social utility, and insofar as infanticide would tend to weaken that socially valuable response, it is, on utilitarian grounds, morally wrong."[39] Feinberg suggests that it is the infant's *similarity* to descriptive persons that makes the consequentialist argument plausible. As he puts it, "It is not potential persons as such who merit our derivative respect but all *near-persons* including higher animals, dead people, infants, and well-developed fetuses, those beings whose similarity to real persons is close enough to render them sacred symbols of the real thing."[40]

Other types of relevant consequences are identified by Engelhardt, who argues for conferred moral standing at birth. On his view, conferred moral standing is justified for those with a social role, and birth is a significant dividing line because it leads to a substantial increase in social role.[41] He argues as follows: "A social role of person can be justified for infants and others in terms of (1) the role's supporting important virtues such as sympathy and care for human life, especially when that life is fragile and defenseless, and

(2) the role's offering a protection against the uncertainties as to when exactly humans become persons strictly, as well as protecting persons during various vicissitudes of competence and incompetence, while (3) in addition securing the important practice of child-rearing through which humans develop as persons in the strict sense."[42]

Finally, Mary Anne Warren points out an additional consequence brought about by conferring moral standing on infants: the desires of many people would be promoted, since most of us care deeply about infants and wish them to be treated well.[43] Warren claims that our attitudes of care and concern increase significantly upon the birth of the child, and in explaining this she too points to the child's social role. It is because infants become involved in social relationships with us that we develop strong psychological bonds toward them.

A second approach to justifying conferred moral standing is contractarian. An example is provided by Green, who advocates the Rawlsian view that morality's function is to furnish a noncoercive means of settling social disputes.[44] The moral rules to be followed are the ones selected in a contractarian choice situation, in which the participants are rational agents who are prevented from having particular information about their own identity and life situation, other than what is common to all participants. On this view, the purpose of morality is to protect the interests of rational agents, and contractors would have a valid reason to confer moral standing on nonrational beings when doing so would prevent harm to the interests of rational agents. Green suggests that in deciding whether to confer moral standing on fetuses, contractors should consider what the consequences for rational agents would be in at least three broad areas: "the effect of conferring or denying rights on our general capacity for sympathy; the effect on the possible interests of particular agents; and, finally, the effect on the character or moral worth of rational agents generally."[45]

Jane English also gives a contractarian argument for conferred moral standing. In discussing the application of Rawls's theory to the moral standing of those who lack descriptive personhood, she states: "Our psychological constitution makes it the case that for our ethical theory to work, it must prohibit certain treatment of non-persons which are significantly person-like. If our moral rules allowed people to treat some person-like non-persons in ways we do not want people to be treated, this would undermine the system of sympathies and attitudes that makes the ethical system work."[46]

It is worth noting that although Green and English use a contractarian framework, their specific arguments for conferred moral standing are consequentialist. This is to be expected, given that the basis of the contractor's decision is an assessment of the overall impact of the decision on the interests of rational agents. Thus, for both the consequentialist and contractarian approaches, arguments for conferred moral standing rest ultimately on consequentialist considerations.

In arguing for conferred moral standing, I shall focus on the consequentialist approach, for several reasons. First, it is more straightforward, in part because it avoids the need to defend the general contractarian moral framework. Furthermore, it does not require defense of a general consequentialist or utilitarian framework, for one can defend decisions on consequentialist grounds without being committed to the general proposition that all morality is reducible to consequentialist considerations. Second, as we have seen, some if not all contractarian approaches to conferred moral standing rely at bottom on consequentialist arguments.

A View on Moral Standing of Embryos, Fetuses, and Infants

A consequentialist approach to conferred moral standing seems promising.[47] However, the version of this approach that has received the most attention — that *birth* is the key factor in determining moral standing — faces several difficulties. First, the view that significant social roles do not begin until birth seems mistaken. Admittedly, the *number* of persons with whom infants have social relationships and the *variety* of those relationships typically increase following birth. However, we should not overlook the fact that the fetus can occupy a social role involving relationships with various individuals. The pregnant woman, for example, can act in ways that promote or detract from the fetus's health. She can attend to the needs of her fetus by avoiding smoking and excessive alcohol use, eating nutritious meals, and seeking treatment for medical problems of her own that can adversely affect the fetus, such as hypertension and diabetes. Also, the psychological attachment of parents to their fetus can be strong. In addition, advances in obstetrical technology have increased our ability to interact with the fetus. Obstetricians can monitor the health of the fetus and provide treatment or early delivery when necessary and feasible. For these reasons, a matrix of social relations between fetus and others is often present well before parturition. Thus, it is difficult to argue that birth constitutes a sharp dividing line between those who should and those who should not have moral standing.

Second, focusing on social role is too narrow an approach. Rather, it is the *overall degree of similarity* that an individual has to the paradigm of descriptive persons — to normal adult human beings — that matters in the consequentialist argument. The reason is that the more similar individuals are to the paradigm, the more likely our ways of treating them will have the kinds of consequences identified by the authors discussed above. Having a social role is not the only possible similarity.

Not all possible similarities are morally relevant, however. For example, although normal adult human beings have two legs, so does the spotted owl, and few would maintain that an owl's having two legs supports the view that normative personhood status should be conferred upon it. It is necessary to identify the *morally relevant* ways in which an individual can be similar to the paradigm. Advocates of the consequentialist approach generally have over-looked the relevance of the criteria of personhood to their argument, for some of these supposed criteria constitute morally relevant ways in which individuals can be similar to descriptive persons. As discussed above, the *potential to cause self-consciousness* has moral relevance because it enters into consequentialist considerations concerning possible future states of affairs involving self-conscious individuals. In addition, the *potential to become self-conscious* is morally relevant not only because it can enter into such consequentialist considerations, but also because the individual with this potential is the same individual — in some sense — as the future self-conscious individual, assuming of course that the potentiality becomes actualized. *Viability* is relevant, in part, because it involves an increase in the fetus's social role. Also, *sentience* is a morally relevant similarity because, as pointed out above, sentience is necessary and sufficient for having moral interests. In addition, *birth* is a morally relevant similarity because typically it results in the infant becoming part of an increasing number and variety of social relationships.

Another similarity not discussed above is a physical resemblance to normal adult human beings. This similarity is morally relevant to the consequentialist argument because, psychologically speaking, we are more likely mentally to associate paradigmatic persons with individuals who *look like* the paradigm than we are to associate them with individuals who do not look like the paradigm. Of course, similarity in physical appearance admits of degrees, and to some extent it is in the eye of the beholder. Nevertheless, it is clear that fetuses near term, for example, are more similar in appearance to the paradigm than embryos are.

To consider the implications of this consequentialist framework based on degrees of similarity, let us begin with infants. We need to ask whether infants are similar enough to the paradigm to give plausibility to the consequentialist argument for conferred moral standing. Are they similar enough to make reasonable the claim that failure to confer a right to life upon them would result in adverse consequences of the sorts mentioned by the various authors discussed above? I would point out that normal infants possess a number of morally relevant similarities with the paradigm: they are *viable, sentient,* have the *potential to become self-conscious,* have been *born,* and are *similar in appearance* to the paradigm of human persons. Although some of these characteristics have been put forward as a sufficient condition for normative personhood of fetuses or infants, none of them by itself constitutes compelling grounds for personhood. What is often overlooked is the significance that should be given to the aggregate possession of these characteristics. The combination of these similarities, I would maintain, is significant enough to warrant conferring upon infants serious moral interests, including a right to life.

Although this conferred personhood status for infants is less secure, resting as it does on consequentialist arguments, than the moral status of descriptive persons, it does not follow that the rights conferred upon them should be regarded as pale, watered-down versions of the rights possessed by descriptive persons. Admittedly, there might be exceptional circumstances in which a conferred right to life conflicts with the right to life of a person in the descriptive sense. In such cases it would be plausible to give priority to the individual who is a descriptive person. Outside of such exceptional cases, however, conferred rights should be regarded as full-bodied. Conferring a serious right to life upon infants might very well promote good consequences of the sorts identified by the authors above. However, it is doubtful that conferring a weak, easily overridden right would have such consequences. Thus, the justification for conferring a right to life is itself undermined if the right conferred is considered a distant cousin to real rights.[48]

Let us consider how this consequentialist framework applies to fetuses and embryos. According to the view I am putting forward, the more similar individuals are to the paradigm, the more likely it is that our ways of treating them will have the kinds of consequences identified. Fetuses early in gestation have fewer similarities to the paradigm than infants do, and embryos have even fewer. As the dissimilarities increase, there remains a possibility of adverse consequences, but the likelihood and magnitude of such consequences diminish. As they diminish, the amount of weight that should be given to these consequentialist considerations decreases. This amounts to saying that the degree of moral consideration that should be given to the individuals decreases. In other words, the degree of conferred moral standing that the individuals should have decreases.

Let us apply these considerations to fetuses that are relatively advanced in development. Such fetuses, assuming they are developmentally normal, possess a number of similarities with the paradigm: they are viable, sentient, possess the potential to become self-conscious, are relatively similar in appearance to descriptive persons, and to some extent occupy a social role.

However, the similarities are slightly less for advanced fetuses than for new-borns because infants typically are more involved in social roles. This suggests that the likelihood and magnitude of adverse consequences that would occur to descriptive persons if advanced fetuses are not treated with respect are slightly less than the likelihood and magnitude of adverse consequences that would occur if infants are not treated with respect. These considerations support the view that advanced fetuses should have a conferred moral status that is close to, but not quite as high as, that of infants. We might say that advanced fetuses should have a conferred right to life, but one that is not quite as strong as that of infants. There might be situations in which an advanced fetus's right to life is overridden by factors that would not be strong enough to override an infant's right to life. Generally, advanced fetuses have serious moral interests that deserve protection, on this view.

I use the expression *relatively advanced in development* to refer to a distinction between fetuses that have a relatively high degree of similarity to the paradigm and fetuses with a lesser degree of similarity. Moreover, I shall use sentience as the characteristic that separates fetuses that are relatively advanced from those that are not as advanced, since sentient and presentient fetuses should be regarded as having different degrees of moral standing, for several reasons. First, because sentience is a morally relevant similarity to the paradigm, the argument for conferred moral standing is stronger for sentient than for nonsentient fetuses. Second, sentience is the basis of moral interests, and we should give greater moral consideration to individuals that have interests than to those that lack interests.

Unfortunately, there is uncertainty concerning when sentience typically begins. Moreover, there likely is variation from one fetus to the next in the gestational age at which it begins. Neurological evidence suggests that typically it could not begin prior to about twenty to twenty-four weeks.[49] However, drawing a sharp line in this gestational age range would not accurately reflect the uncertainty involved. It is better to acknowledge that there is a gray area in which it is uncertain as to whether a given fetus is sentient. By contrast, normal fetuses closer to term are reasonably regarded as sentient.

In applying the consequentialist framework to the early postconception period, we obtain very different results. For preembryos, the argument for conferred moral standing is weak because they lack viability, sentience, a social role, any physical resemblance to descriptive persons, and the potential to become self-conscious. They have very little similarity to the paradigm, and it is implausible to argue that failure to accord them a right to life would have adverse consequences of the sorts described above. However, conferring a minor degree of moral status upon them is justifiable because they have the potential to cause self-consciousness and might therefore be regarded by some as a symbol of descriptive persons.

Similar remarks can be made concerning the embryo proper, which lacks viability, sentience, a social role, and physical resemblance to descriptive persons. Because there is so little similarity with the paradigm, the likelihood and magnitude of adverse consequences that would occur to descriptive persons if embryos are not given a right to life are low. Therefore, the degree of moral consideration that should be given to them is small, compared, say, to advanced fetuses. However, embryos are slightly more similar to the paradigm than preembryos because they have the potential to become self-conscious. Thus, it is reasonable to hold that we should confer slightly more moral status upon them than we confer on preembryos.

Finally, presentient fetuses occupy an intermediate position. They have the potential to become self-conscious, and to some extent they can occupy a social role. However, the degree of dissimilarity with the paradigm, together with the fact that as nonsentient creatures they lack moral interests of their own, suggests that a conferred right to life would not be justifiable. Nevertheless, some degree of moral consideration would seem warranted, based on their limited similarity to descriptive persons. This implies, for example, that abortion of a presentient fetus is an act having some degree of moral import, and that some reasons for abortion might be morally too trivial to justify it. Moreover, as the presentient period progresses, the fetus becomes more similar in appearance to the paradigm. This justifies giving greater consideration to fetuses near sentience than to those in an earlier presentient period.

This consequentialist approach helps explain why it is reasonable to hold that moral status increases as the offspring develops during pregnancy. Not only does the conceptus become more developed, but there are certain milestones along the way that represent morally relevant similarities with normal adult human beings. As these milestones like sentience and birth are achieved, the likelihood and magnitude of the adverse consequences of not treating the individual with consideration increase. The presence of such milestones is at odds with the view that moral standing increases linearly as pregnancy progresses.

Objections and Responses

An objection might be raised to my view concerning fetuses with relatively advanced development. As Warren has stated, "It is impossible to treat fetuses *in utero* as if they were persons without treating women as if they were something less than persons. The extension of equal rights to sentient fetuses would inevitably license severe violations of women's basic rights to personal autonomy and physical security."[50] Although my view does not confer equal rights on advanced fetuses, it confers rights that are substantial enough that concerns like Warren's might be raised. The concern is that such conferred status might justify violating women's rights, as in forcing pregnant women to undergo unwanted treatment for the sake of the fetus or prosecuting women for behavior harmful to the fetus. In reply, assuming that advanced fetuses have the moral status I suggest, it does not automatically follow that it is morally justifiable to coerce women to undergo invasive medical procedures for the sake of the fetus or to prosecute them for harmful behavior. Moreover, because women have full moral standing but advanced fetuses do not, there should be a presumption in favor of the woman's interests when conflicts arise. Thus, although coercive maternal treatment might be warranted in a very limited range of situations, the wholesale violation of the rights and liberty of pregnant women envisioned by Warren would not be justifiable. The implications of my view for maternal-fetal conflicts will be discussed in greater detail in Chapter 9.

Another objection focuses on a weakness of consequentialist arguments. It might be claimed, for example, that there is too much uncertainty to predict reliably that adverse consequences would follow from failure to confer significant rights on infants. Although uncertainty sometimes is a decisive consideration against consequentialist arguments,[51] it is less compelling in the present context. To see this, we need only consider what would be involved in not conferring a right to life upon infants and others who are very similar to persons in the descriptive sense. If infants and others who lack self-consciousness because of severe mental retardation, senility, or other debilitation were regarded as not having a right to life, then the proscription against killing them would be removed. Not only would individuals in those categories be in jeopardy, but so would individuals who border on those categories. Persons in the descriptive sense would reasonably feel threatened in this situation, for several reasons. First, they might be concerned that those they care about—infants of their own or loved ones who have become senile, for example—might be killed, or at least that efforts to keep them alive might be weakened. Second, they might be concerned that they could become debilitated some day, perhaps becoming borderline cases, and therefore be at risk themselves. These sorts of fears would cause anxiety and, in some cases, deeper suffering for descriptive persons. The overall level of security for descriptive persons would be diminished. Thus, some of the predicted undesirable consequences would unavoidably arise from a policy of not conferring normative personhood on infants and others who are highly similar to the paradigm. These considerations support the consequentialist framework I have put forward.

The Procreator's Duty to Offspring

The view concerning moral standing defended above has implications concerning the obligations of procreators toward their offspring. It is important to include discussion of such obligations in our ethical framework. However, a comprehensive account is not needed, for purposes of this book. The reason is that the *rearing* of one's genetic offspring is classified as an aspect of procreation, as I argued in Chapter 1. A comprehensive discussion of procreator's obligations would address rearing duties, but issues pertaining to the postnatal rearing of children are not included in this book.

The relevant topic is the obligations that procreators, and potential procreators, have before and during gestation. These include any duties that procreators might have toward preembryos, embryos, and fetuses, as well as duties that exist before and during gestation to future children. I believe that this topic can be addressed in terms of an obligation to act beneficently toward the offspring. This includes one of the obligations identified by Winston and mentioned at the beginning of this chapter: an obligation to protect the offspring from harm.[52] An expanded statement of this obligation is provided by Deborah Mathieu, who points out that procreators have a duty to refrain from causing harm to offspring and, to some extent, to try to prevent and remove harm.[53]

This obligation to act beneficently is mediated by the fetus's moral status. In general terms, the greater the moral status, the greater the strength of the obligation. When the fetus has a significant conferred moral standing, as in the case of fetuses that are relatively advanced in development, the pregnant woman has a relatively strong obligation to act beneficently toward it. This implies, among other things, that abortion on demand is not ethically justifiable in regard to such fetuses.

On the other hand, early in gestation, when the fetus or embryo does not have a significant moral standing, we would describe the pregnant woman's obligation somewhat differently. If she intends to carry the fetus to term, then she has an obligation to the possible future child to act beneficently toward the fetus. However, she can choose to end this obligation by having an abortion. If the woman does not intend to carry the fetus to term, then because embryos and early fetuses have a relatively low moral status, her obligation to act beneficently is very weak and her decision to end the pregnancy is ethically justifiable.

4

Assigning Priorities

The issues to be discussed in Part 2 of this book can be characterized as conflicts of ethical values. To be useful in addressing those issues, our ethical framework must include an acceptable approach to assigning priorities to conflicting values.

In the Introduction, I stated that there is generally a presumption in favor of autonomy, and in Chapters 1 and 2, I identified reasons for a presumption favoring freedom to procreate and freedom not to procreate. The value conflicts that arise in reproductive ethics almost always involve conflicts between reproductive freedom and other values. Some of these conflicts will be resolved by appealing to the presumption in favor of reproductive freedom, but a major challenge posed by issues in reproductive ethics is to decide when reproductive freedom should be overridden by other values. One might even say that this is the central question in reproductive ethics. The purpose of an ethical framework, essentially, is to help provide a reasoned approach to answering this question.

Ethical Values

Perhaps I should explain more fully what I mean by "ethical values." I use the term broadly, to include appeals to all the ethical principles, rules, and concerns relevant to reproductive ethics. Certain ethical values are central to the topic of reproductive ethics and were discussed in Chapters 1–3: freedom to procreate and freedom not to procreate; the moral consideration that should be given to fetuses, which varies depending on the degree of similarity with the paradigm of descriptive persons; and the rights and interests of infants, based on their conferred moral standing. In the Introduction, I identified a number of additional ethical values relevant to reproductive ethics. To highlight the fact that there are many relevant values, let us briefly consider some of the main ways in which values are expressed, as listed below.

Middle-level ethical principles. Ethical values include the concerns expressed in middle-level ethical principles. These include the principles of autonomy, beneficence, nonmaleficence, and justice.[1] These principles are called middle-level because they are less general and comprehensive than ethical theories, such as utilitarianism and Kantianism, but more general than rules.

Moral rules. Ethical values also include the concerns expressed by moral rules. Examples of moral rules include: Don't cause pain; don't deceive; and don't cheat.[2] The Ten Commandments provide additional examples.

Respect for persons. An important value is respect for persons. Those who are persons in the descriptive sense deserve respect because of their special capacities, which include the abilities to deliberate rationally, choose values and goals, and carry out plans in pursuit of their goals. Respecting persons includes respecting their capacities to do these things. In addition, there are conditions that are necessary for, or at least facilitate, a person's exercise of these capacities. These include being alive, maintaining one's bodily integrity, and being free to make choices and act upon them.[3] Showing respect for persons also requires refraining from eliminating or diminishing these conditions.

Rights. Respect for persons in the descriptive sense requires respect for their rights. However, appeals to rights cannot simply be equated with respect for descriptive persons. The reason is that there are individuals who are not persons in the descriptive sense but who justifiably are regarded as having rights because they have the conferred moral standing of normative personhood. A number of rights are especially relevant to reproductive ethics and medical ethics generally. These include the right not to be killed, the right to bodily self-determination, and the right of confidentiality, among others.

Consequences. One of the central ideas of moral philosophy is that consequences are relevant to the rightness and wrongness of actions. Good consequences are to be valued, but the question of what sorts of consequences are most important has been debated at length. Hedonistic utilitarian theories equate good consequences with the happiness or pleasure of persons. Other views equate it with the satisfaction of rational preferences, and yet others with the objective well-being of persons. For our purposes, it will not be necessary to compare critically these different versions of consequentialism.[4]

Role-related duties. Values also are expressed in statements of duty. Role-related duties that are especially relevant to our topic include the duties of health care providers, such as the physician's duties to protect confidentiality and obtain informed consent. They also include the duties of procreators toward their offspring, a main one for our purposes being a duty of beneficence toward offspring.[5] Of course, moral duties other than role-related ones can be pertinent to reproductive ethics. These are general duties that we owe to all persons, regardless of our roles in relation to them, such as the duty to avoid killing, to avoid harming, and so on. Nevertheless, it is worth highlighting role-specific duties because they are relevant so frequently.[6]

Virtues. Virtues pertain to the moral character of persons; they are characteristics of persons that constitute moral excellences. Virtues that seem especially relevant to reproductive ethics include honesty, compassion, and integrity.[7] Honesty is the virtue of being truthful. Compassion involves acting in ways that attempt to remove or diminish the suffering or losses of others. Closely related to compassion is the concept of "caring." Some have argued that more attention should be given to an ethics of caring, in which feelings of a beneficent sort and concern about interpersonal relationships motivate behavior.[8] To have integrity is to stand firm in one's personal values. People have personal values that reflect their views of the good life, their religious beliefs, goals they wish to pursue, and preferences of various sorts. Of particular relevance, integrity includes refusals to perform actions based on conscientious objection. Although virtues pertain to moral character, they can be relevant to the evaluation of actions; the fact that an action is required by a certain virtue can be a reason supporting it.

These different ways of expressing values are not mutually exclusive. For example, respect for persons requires respect for their rights. Similarly, certain rules, such as "Risks should be balanced by benefits," express in specific ways the content of the broader principle of beneficence. Other rules express the principle of autonomy, such as "Competent patients have a right to refuse treatment." We should not be troubled by the fact that these ways of expressing values overlap. The important thing is to take into account all of the many ethical values that are pertinent.

The Inadequacy of Traditional Theories

It might be claimed that we should resolve value conflicts by using one of the traditional ethical theories, such as utilitarianism, Kantianism, natural law theory, or contractualism. However, many ethicists who have spent considerable time providing ethics consultations in the clinical setting have come to the view that these traditional theories are not suitable for resolving concrete ethical dilemmas. The conceptual shortcomings of these theories already were widely understood, but clinical ethics brought to light their inadequacy at the practical level. Specifically, these traditional theories provide little help when it comes to assigning priorities to conflicting ethical values in the context of specific cases and issues in medical ethics.[9]

Because the shortcomings of these theories are widely recognized, I shall discuss only briefly their inability to assign priorities to conflicting ethical values, focusing on what I take to be the leading contenders among the traditional theories: utilitarianism in its various forms, Kantianism, and contractualism. Although some ethical theories are theological in nature, in this book I focus on nontheological ones.

RULE AND ACT UTILITARIANISM

Let us consider how rule utilitarianism would attempt to resolve conflicting ethical values.[10] Rule utilitarians would seek to adopt, as a policy for dealing with a type of conflict, that rule or set of rules the implementation of which would maximize utility. This involves identifying, as possible policies, the alternative rules or sets of rules for dealing with the type of conflict in question. Then the likely consequences of implementing each alternative policy should be considered, and the one that seems most likely to maximize utility should be selected. The ethically correct solution to a particular case involving that type of conflict would be obtained by applying the utility-maximizing policy to that case. The problem, which becomes apparent once one attempts to apply this approach in the clinical setting, is that usually there are a number of alternative policies and we cannot reasonably predict which one would maximize expected utility. Thus, rule utilitarianism typically is unhelpful in resolving such conflicts.

Utilitarians are accustomed to this objection and have a standard reply. They acknowledge that often there is not as much information available as one would like for making predictions and that estimates of expected utilities will sometimes be inaccurate. However, they point out that utilitarianism only requires that we do the best we can — that we try to obtain the most reasonable estimates of expected utilities given the available data. The utilitarians assure us that, even though data is limited, common sense and thoughtful deliberation will enable us to arrive at defensible estimates of expected utilities.

Unfortunately, this reply seriously underestimates the difficulties in calculating and comparing expected utilities in the clinical setting. The problem is that the medical and psychosocial dimensions of typical clinical dilemmas are sufficiently complex and uncertain that usually we do not even have enough data to construct defensible best guesses concerning which policy would maximize expected utility. To illustrate this problem, let us consider one of the issues in reproductive ethics — maternal refusal of treatment needed for the sake of the fetus — and let us interpret utility as happiness. Various policies could be adopted for dealing with such cases. One policy would require administering the necessary treatment in all cases; this would involve always giving priority to fetal well-being. A second policy would require always respecting the mother's refusal, giving priority to maternal autonomy. A third approach would involve treating in selected cases, based on additional factors to be identified.

A utilitarian might argue that a policy of always treating would maximize happiness, since treatments might be life-saving for the fetus, and sometimes even for the mother, and might prevent handicaps for the newborn. Thus, by maximizing the probability of disease-free survival for fetuses and mothers, this policy would give them the greatest opportunity for future happiness. However, there are a number of considerations that make this prediction questionable. To begin, there is considerable uncertainty concerning the degree to which lives would be saved and neonatal handicaps prevented by such obstetric interventions. Also, one would have to take into account a possible disruption of the doctor-patient relationship resulting from forcing the woman to undergo treatment. Such a disruption could harm her, especially if it caused her to become unwilling to cooperate with care providers during the remainder of her hospitalization. One also would need to consider the possible effects of the policy upon doctor-patient relationships generally. Women might become less inclined to trust their obstetricians or seek prenatal care, and these consequences could be harmful to patients and fetuses. Another consideration is the possible brutalizing effect upon caregivers. Coercing patients might tend to make caregivers less sensitive to the rights of pregnant women, and this could adversely affect future patients. The rule utilitarian who advocates always treating assumes that the potential harm to fetuses and pregnant women due to disruption of relationships and brutalizing effects is less than the harm to fetuses and pregnant women due to withholding needed treatments. Furthermore, for each policy a rule utilitarian might defend, there would be a similar assumption concerning a comparison of harms. However, medical and sociological data are not available to support these various assumptions. Because each argument could be criticized for its unsupported assumptions, there would be no rational basis for deciding among them. In such a context, appeals to common sense in support of a given policy might well be speculative, rather than defensible argumentation. The reason is that the assumptions in question depend on uncertain medical outcomes, psychological responses of the persons involved, and long-term interpersonal relations of many individuals. These medical and psychosocial dimensions of the problem of estimating expected utilities are too complex to be resolved easily by common sense.

Act utilitarianism faces similar problems. Rather than focusing on policies, the act utilitarian would have us choose the option in each case that maximizes happiness. However, the medical and psychosocial dimensions of such cases are sufficiently complex, as illustrated by the above discussion, that our state of knowledge does not permit defensible predictions of the consequences of the various options with regard to the happiness of the relevant people.[11]

These problems concerning utilitarian calculations are not only a feature of the type of conflict I have been discussing but arise in the attempted application of rule- and act utilitarianism to ethical dilemmas in reproductive and perinatal medicine generally. Moreover, they arise whether one equates utility with happiness or uses the other interpretations of utility, such as pleasure or the satisfaction of rational desires.

KANTIANISM

Kant's theory of ethics places constraints on the pursuit of good consequences. Central to his theory is the idea that we should treat other persons always as ends in themselves and never as means only.[12] This principle, referred to as the *categorical imperative,* is never to be violated, even if doing so is necessary to bring about good consequences.

A major difficulty concerns how to apply this principle when one has conflicting duties to two or more parties and cannot treat all the affected individuals as ends in themselves. To illustrate this problem, we might consider situations in which a duty to prevent harm to a specific individual conflicts with a duty to respect the autonomy of another. Examples include cases in which parents refuse aggressive life-preserving treatment for children with serious birth injuries. In some cases of this type, withholding treatment will be harmful to the child. In order to treat such children as ends in themselves, physicians in such cases should attempt to provide the needed therapies, perhaps by seeking a court order if necessary.[13] In following this approach the physician would honor the duty to prevent harm to the child. However, in order to treat the parents as ends in themselves, the physician would be required to respect their autonomy. Taking the decision from their hands would especially undermine parental autonomy if the decision were likely to have a major impact on their lives, as would happen if the survival of a handicapped child were likely to affect the family in major ways. If we had to rely solely on Kantianism to resolve such cases, we would be at an impasse, with no basis for deciding which of the parties should be treated as ends in themselves. This type of problem presents a serious difficulty in the application of Kant's theory. In putting forward the categorical imperative in *Foundations of the Metaphysics of Morals,* Kant did not consider situations in which the imperative poses conflicting obligations toward two or more individuals, much less address the question of how his theory would deal with such cases.

One might consider whether an answer is provided in another major work of Kant's on ethics, *The Metaphysics of Morals,* in which he further develops his theory of moral duties and attempts to show how various duties can be derived from the categorical imperative.[14] Situations that I have characterized as involving conflicting duties are described by Kant as involving conflicting grounds of obligation.[15] Although he acknowledges that there can be conflicting grounds of obligation, in this book too there is no discussion of how to resolve such conflicts. His objectives are primarily theoretical; he wants to show that indeed we are justified in believing that we have certain moral duties, by demonstrating how those duties can be derived from the fundamental principles set forth in *Foundations of the Metaphysics of Morals.*[16] Furthermore, to my knowledge no adequate answer to the problem of conflicting duties is found in any of the other ethical writings of Kant, nor has any commentator satisfactorily resolved the problem of how Kant's theory might handle such conflicts.[17]

CONTRACTUALISM

Contractarian theory has received much attention since the publication of *A Theory of Justice* by John Rawls.[18] It might be asked whether Rawls's contractarian approach could be applied to issues in practical ethics. Even if we put aside conceptual problems with Rawls's theory, however, we find that it is not very helpful in resolving issues in clinical ethics. In fairness to Rawls, it is doubtful that such a task was one of his objectives in writing his book. His theory aims, rather, at identifying and justifying general principles of justice upon which the structure of a society may be founded. The theory would have to be developed considerably in order to provide answers about bioethics in a broad range of cases. Whether this can be done remains to be seen.

I am aware of only one contractarian theory that attempts to provide a method for resolving individual cases, that of Robert M. Veatch.[19] He proposes a triple-contract theory in which decisions are based on the results of three contract situations. The first is a social contract establishing the most basic ethical principles for human interaction. The contractors would attempt to take the moral point of view, in that the welfare of other persons is considered on the same scale as one's own. They also should try to approximate the qualities of the ideal observer, who is omniscient, sensitive, impartial, dispassionate, and consistent. There would be no selection of contractors; rather, the contract situation would be open to all, so that in a sense the entire moral community would come together. Veatch believes that the main principles that would actually be chosen include beneficence, autonomy, truth telling, promise keeping, justice, and avoiding killing.

In the second contract situation, the community of lay people negotiates with the medical profession. The purpose of the contract is to establish the role-specific duties of physicians. These duties must be consistent with the basic principles agreed to in the first contract. Again, participants attempt to approximate as best they can the moral point of view and the ideal observer. The third contract is to be negotiated between the individual physician and patient. Its purpose is to reach agreement on moral dimensions of the professional-client relationship left as matters of choice by the first and second contracts. It could, for example, address the patient's wishes concerning access to information. Any agreement reached must be consistent with the first two contracts.

Of particular relevance is Veatch's discussion of assigning priorities to conflicting ethical principles. He argues for a lexical ordering according to which the nonconsequentialist principles as a group take priority over beneficence, which he defines as the principle "of producing good for one another."[20] The nonconsequentialist principles are considered coequal, and conflicts between them are to be handled by a "balancing strategy": we should opt for the course of action producing, on balance, the lesser violation of nonconsequentialist principles. This balancing is to be carried out in the contract situation. Empirical studies would be relevant, to eliminate options which "involve more than a necessary amount of infringement on the basic principles."[21] Taking into account such information, actual contractors would strive to assume the moral point of view and try to balance the conflicting principles.

Unfortunately, this approach is not very helpful in practice, in part because the concept of "lesser violation of the nonconsequentialist principles" is vague, and Veatch provides little guidance concerning how he would apply it. As Veatch points out himself, this method "is probably not a very satisfying one," in that it "does not provide a precise measuring technique permitting the balancing of counterclaims."[22] Another difficulty is that ethical conflicts in medicine frequently are between nonconsequentialist principles and the consequentialist principle that one should prevent harm to others. Examples of issues involving this type of conflict include parents refusing medically needed treatment for their children, psychiatric patients threatening to harm others, and pregnant women refusing treatment needed for the sake of the fetus.

Unfortunately, Veatch's theory is unclear concerning this type of conflict. He might intend such cases to be handled by his lexical ordering, but this would give implausible results, since it implies that the liberty of persons should never be circumscribed to prevent harm to others. What is usually referred to as the *harm principle* would thus be rejected. Perhaps he intends such conflicts to be resolved by choosing the "lesser overall violation," but again this is too vague to be helpful. Ethical problems often arise precisely because it is not clear which option would involve the lesser overall violation of the conflicting principles. Thus, Veatch's theory, in its current state of development at least, does not resolve the problem of assigning priorities to conflicting principles. It seems, then, that no contractarian approach put forward to date is helpful in making decisions about value conflicts in reproductive and perinatal medicine.

We have seen that the leading contenders among traditional ethical theories fail to resolve the problem of assigning priorities to conflicting ethical values. In pointing this out, however, I do not mean to imply that these theories lack worth or that they should be completely abandoned. On the contrary, each of them is valuable in part because it identifies certain ethical values that should be taken into account. For example, utilitarian theories remind us of the ethical relevance of the consequences of our actions, insofar as these are good or bad, and Kantianism underscores the importance of respect for persons. Nevertheless, the inability of traditional theories to provide practical guidance suggests that we must look elsewhere.

Assigning Priorities: Four Ways

In resolving value conflicts, one unavoidably makes assumptions concerning how to go about the task of assigning priorities. In effect, these assumptions involve choosing from among several approaches to assigning priorities. In this section, I identify the main approaches that can be taken and argue in support of one of them. It is important to consider these alternative approaches because their selection affects the decisions made in individual cases.

To identify these approaches, we need to consider the following question, one that often is not dealt with explicitly in discussions of ethics: At what level of generality should the assigning of priorities to conflicting ethical values be made? When we attempt to answer this question, we see that there are four main possibilities:

1. The prioritization is considered to hold *whenever* the values in question conflict.
2. The prioritization is made in the context of a certain issue or type of case.

The prioritization is considered to hold for all cases of that type. The same prioritization would not necessarily hold in other types of cases in which the values in question conflict.

3. The prioritization is made in the context of individual cases and might differ in different cases of a given type.

4. For some issues or types of cases, the prioritization takes place in the context of individual cases, as in approach 3, and for other issues or types of cases the prioritization is considered to hold for all cases of that type, as in approach 2.

The first approach involves assigning a hierarchical ranking, or lexical order, to values or groups of values. Once the ranking is made, it is fixed, and it is applied to all cases without exception. An example of this approach is Veatch's lexical ordering, in which a group of nonconsequentialist principles always takes priority over the principle of beneficence.[23] An example specifically in reproductive and perinatal medicine is the view that Joseph Fletcher puts forward in *The Ethics of Genetic Control*.[24] On his view, one always should choose the act that is likely best to promote the well-being of the greatest number of persons. In other words, the overall well-being of all affected persons is always the highest-ranked value.

The difficulty with this first approach is that it fails to deal adequately with the complexity of morality. For any given value or set of values that supposedly is ranked first, we can always think of a situation in which that value or set of values is overridden by other values. With regard to Veatch's lexical ordering, for example, there are situations in which the principle of beneficence — and, more specifically, the principle that we should prevent harm to others — takes priority over the nonconsequentialist principle of autonomy.[25] The problem with Fletcher's ordering of values is that sometimes respect for persons should override good consequences.

According to the second approach, a ranking is assigned that holds for all cases in which a given issue arises. To illustrate, consider the issue of whether to carry out requests by single women for artificial insemination, in which a main conflict is between the reproductive freedom of the woman requesting artificial insemination and, arguably, prevention of harm to the child who would be produced. The view that this issue should be resolved by always giving priority to prevention of supposed harms to the child — and hence that requests for artificial insemination by single women should never be honored — is an example of the approach in question. For each issue, it identifies a preferable value (or set of values) and assigns priority to the chosen value(s) in every case in which the issue arises.

Although its inflexibility would seem to be a weakness, this type of approach is commonly encountered in discussions of reproductive and perinatal ethics. It is exemplified by those who assert the following familiar views, among others: surrogate motherhood should never be permitted; abortion is always wrong; forced maternal treatment should never be carried out; and the interests of handicapped newborns should always prevail over the interests of their families. The difficulty with this approach is similar to that of the first approach. Even if we restrict ourselves to a particular issue, the view that a certain ethical value, or set of values, should always have priority often reflects an oversimplified picture of the moral situation. For a given value or set of values that supposedly is ranked first for a particular issue, often we can think of a case of the type in question in which that value or set of values is overridden by other moral considerations.

The third approach seeks, for every issue, a ranking of ethical values in the context of each specific case. It acknowledges each of the main conflicting ethical values involved in a given issue, and it seeks a balancing or compromise of those values. This might involve giving priority to one value (or group of values) in one subset of cases but assigning priority to a different value (or group of values) in another subset of cases.[26] The decision concerning how to rank the values in a given case involves two main elements. First, for each issue, it requires the identification of morally relevant factors that can vary in degree from one case to the next. Second, it gives careful consideration to the degree to which the various factors are present in the case at hand and bases the decision on the extent to which they are present.

To illustrate this approach, consider the issue of when it is justifiable for physicians to recommend aggressive treatment following detection of fetal anomalies. Modern obstetrics makes possible a number of interventions that, in certain situations, could potentially benefit the fetus, including labor-arresting drugs, cesarean section for fetal indications, and in some cases surgical fetal therapy. Although decisions about such interventions rest with the pregnant woman, the role of the obstetrician includes counseling her and making recommendations when appropriate. In such situations, obstetricians are faced with the question of when it is ethically justifiable to recommend aggressive interventions for the sake of the fetus. Because procedures that potentially are therapeutic for the fetus often involve risks to the pregnant woman, the decision concerning what to recommend frequently involves a conflict between maternal and fetal well-being. Morally relevant factors that can vary from one case to the next include fetal prognosis, the reliability of the fetal diagnosis, the degree of maternal harm that could occur in a given procedure, the likelihood that such harm would occur, the degree of benefit the procedure promises for the fetus, and the likelihood that such benefit would occur. According to the approach in question, the decision would be made by weighing the morally relevant factors pertaining to maternal well-being against those pertaining to fetal well-being. Thus, the lower the magnitude and probability of harms to the woman and the greater the magnitude and probability of benefits to the fetus, the stronger the argument for recommending aggressive intervention. In some cases, high maternal risks and low potential fetal benefits would lead to a recommendation of nonintervention. In other cases, low maternal risks and potentially high fetal benefits would result in a recommendation for aggressive treatment.

Although the third approach avoids rankings that hold for all cases in which a given issue arises, it leaves open the possibility of a strong presumption in favor of certain ethical values. To illustrate, consider the issue of forced maternal treatment during pregnancy. One possible view is that forced maternal treatment is ethically justifiable only in rare, exceptional circumstances. This view, which almost always gives priority to maternal autonomy over fetal well-being, is consistent with the third approach.

This third approach is a type of casuistic reasoning. Recent work by Jonsen and Toulmin has rekindled interest in casuistry and raised awareness of its usefulness in clinical ethics.[27] Casuistry is a method of justifying decisions about what to do in specific cases, and it has several distinguishing features. First, it is not an ethical theory in the sense in which utilitarianism, Kantianism, and contractarianism are theories. That is, it attempts neither a comprehensive account of ethics nor an account of the "ultimate" grounding of ethical decisions. Second, it is not a deductive approach. It does not "apply" principles to cases in the sense of attempting to deduce conclusions from premises consisting of ethical principles and factual descriptions of cases. Rather, it is a case-based approach in which argument proceeds by comparing the case at hand with other cases of similar type. Usually, at some point the argument includes comparisons with paradigm cases, in which it is reasonably clear what course of action should be taken. Third, the comparisons of cases are made in terms of the *morally relevant factors,* of which I gave examples above, and which can vary in magnitude from case to case. The decision that is best will depend on the extent to which these factors are present in the given case. Because it will be helpful to have a term to refer to the morally relevant factors that arise in casuistic reasoning, I shall call them *casuistic factors.*[28] Fourth, casuistry does not generally claim to reach certainty in its conclusions. The strength of the conclusions depends on the plausibility of the comparisons with the paradigm cases. In casuistic argumentation, there is room for disagreement concerning such matters as whether a case is more similar to one or another paradigm, and whether the casuistic factors are present in a case to sufficient degree to warrant a given conclusion. When such disagreements cannot be resolved, it might sometimes be appropriate to conclude that several alternative courses of action are permissible, or that casuistry does not provide an answer in that case.[29]

There are pros and cons to this third approach. Its advantages include the fact that it avoids the oversimplification of the first two approaches. Also, it reflects better how decision making in bioethics usually does and should take place. It does this by taking into account a common characteristic of ethical issues that arise in the clinical setting — variation among cases. For a given type of conflict, there usually are a number of morally relevant ways in which instances of it can vary from one situation to another, and these variations can make a difference in the decision that ought to be made in a given case. On the other hand, although this approach is more flexible than the first two, it nevertheless falls short of the degree of flexibility that is desirable in dealing with the complexities of bioethics. Although generally cases should be decided individually, it is possible that for some issues there might be compelling reasons to prioritize similarly in all cases. For example, in Chapter 5 I shall argue that, based on broad concerns about positive eugenics, physicians should refuse all requests for prenatal genetic testing for nondisease characteristics, such as intelligence, height, or body build, rather than deciding on a case-by-case basis. The third approach does not seem amenable to this type of broad critical assessment of an issue.

The fourth approach is preferable to the third because, although it recognizes the importance of case-by-case decision making generally, it also acknowledges that for some issues there might be broad social considerations that provide reasons for adopting a uniform policy across all cases. Thus, it leaves room for such broad considerations to be taken into account. Moreover, the fourth approach does not commit one to the view that at least some prioritizations must be made at the level of issues; rather, it simply leaves open that possibility. It holds that there is a presumption in favor of prioritizing in the context of individual cases, but that this presumption might sometimes be overridden. Thus, the fourth approach enables us to grapple with the "big picture" — to ask where we are going and where we should be going with respect to human reproduction — and to formulate policies that are capable of taking into account the big picture.

Because the fourth approach includes the type of reasoning involved in the third approach, it too is casuistic. It will be helpful to have terms to distinguish these two versions of casuistry. Therefore, I shall refer to the third approach as the *strict* casuistic approach and to the fourth as the *modified* casuistic approach.

Objections and Responses

Currently, there is great interest in exploring the merits and problems of casuistry. One objection, put forward by Kevin Wm. Wildes, is that casuistry is possible only if there is a commonly agreed-upon morality. Roman Catholic moral theology provided a common morality that served as the context for casuistry during its heyday in the Middle Ages. By contrast, modern secular society is characterized by a plurality of moral viewpoints.[30] Wildes claims that casuistry needs a common morality because otherwise there cannot be agreement concerning paradigm cases. Wildes's claims are seriously mistaken. Although some shared assumptions are needed for casuistry to work, what is required is much less than Wildes asserts. There must be agreement concerning the ethical values held to be relevant to cases. Also, there is a need for agreement in moral judgments concerning the paradigm cases used. This level of agreement seems possible, even with modern pluralism. People of diverse moral communities generally accept the main ethical values of secular bioethics, such as beneficence, autonomy, nonmaleficence, and fairness. Moreover, agreement over paradigms need not hold for every case we attempt to resolve, but only often enough for casuistry to be generally helpful. This level of agreement is sufficient to search for reasonable decisions within a casuistic framework, although it does not constitute the high level of moral consensus that apparently surrounded the use of casuistry during the Middle Ages.

Another objection, voiced by John D. Arras, is that casuistry cannot achieve consensus on all issues.[31] Arras points to issues concerning which our society seems unable to reach consensus, such as abortion and justice in health care delivery — that is, the degree to which health care should be made available, at public expense, to those unable to afford it. He asserts that casuists claim that their method will result in consensus concerning such issues, but they cannot deliver. In response, Arras greatly overestimates the ambitions of casuistry and places unreasonable demands upon it. Casuists neither seek nor expect society-wide consensus concerning all conclusions reached by casuistic argumentation. Casuistry could be described as seeking conclusions that are hypothetical rather than categorical: they are reasonable *if* one accepts certain assumptions about ethical values and paradigm cases. Moreover, we should simply recognize that a general consensus concerning all controversial moral issues is not possible. To fault a method of ethical reasoning for its inability to deliver such a consensus is to use a standard that is too severe.

Arras also claims that because casuistry takes intuitions about cases as a given, it is not able to examine those intuitions critically. Because of this, he says, casuistry cannot challenge established social views or the values of the male-dominated medical profession.[32] Although this seems to be a valid criticism, it is aimed primarily at what I have called the strict casuistic approach. By contrast, the modified casuistic approach allows the introduction of broad social considerations, including ways in which the power structure in medicine influences accepted views. In being open to such considerations, it is able critically to assess intuitions about cases, making possible the rejection of previously held intuitions when there are adequate reasons for doing so. Thus, it does not preclude the critical assessment of established views as strict casuistry seems to do, and it is not subject to the objection in question.

Casuistry also has been criticized by Tom Tomlinson, who claims that alternative sets of paradigm cases could be chosen and that different paradigms result in different conclusions.[33] He illustrates his argument by using an example of casuistic reasoning that I put forward in "Justification in Ethics."[34] The case I presented for resolution involved an obstetrical patient who was a Jehovah's Witness. She was diagnosed to have abruptio placenta (premature separation of the placenta from the uterus) and agreed to a medically indicated cesarean section. After delivery, she developed blood coagulation problems resulting in the need for a life-saving blood transfusion, which she refused. Her husband worked as a manual laborer, earning a modest income, and the family also was receiving welfare assistance. The patient and her husband were raising six children, including the newborn infant. If the patient were to die, only one other family member, a grandmother, would be available to help care for the newborn and other children. The physicians were faced with two options: respect the patient's refusal of treatment, allowing her to die; or seek a court order to administer transfusions on the grounds of preventing harm to the dependent children.

According to the casuistic approach I proposed in that article (and continue to advocate), for each alternative course of action, one should try to identify a paradigm case in which that course of action would be the ethically preferable one. Then one should compare the case at hand with the paradigm cases, using the casuistic factors as the basis of comparison. If the case under consideration is closer to one paradigm than to the others, then the course of action justifiable in that paradigm would also be justifiable in the case at hand. In applying this approach to the Jehovah's Witness case, I sought a paradigm case for each of the two options facing the physicians. For a paradigm in which the patient's wishes should be overruled, I described a second case involving refusal of life-saving blood transfusions by a Jehovah's Witness. In that case, also, there were dependent children, and the family circumstances made it likely that a relatively great amount of harm would befall the children if the patient died. I also described a paradigm case in which the patient's wishes should be respected.

This third case, too, involved a Jehovah's Witness refusing life-saving transfusions. In this case, however, the family situation was much different. Because there was an extended family capable of helping raise the children and the family was financially secure, much less harm was likely to occur to the children as a result of the patient's death. A comparison of the case to be resolved with the paradigms showed it to be more similar to the second case than to the third, yielding a conclusion that a court order should be sought in the case at hand.

Tomlinson suggests that there is an equally satisfactory set of paradigm cases that would lead to a different conclusion. Specifically, he asks us to consider a case in which a mother refuses to donate a kidney to her child who needs a kidney transplant. Tomlinson points out that it would be wrong to force the woman to donate a kidney, and he claims that this paradigm, when applied to the blood transfusion case, supports a decision not to seek a court order. However, this conclusion does not follow. To see this, we need only consider what happens when we replace my paradigm case for not seeking a court order with Tomlinson's. Now we are comparing the case at hand to my second case and Tomlinson's case. In terms of the casuistic factors, the case at hand is closer to my second case, for several reasons: the risks of removing a kidney are much greater than the risks of giving life-saving blood to someone; the potential harms to the pediatric renal patient can possibly be avoided by means other than performing the contemplated procedure on the mother; and a transplant might not be successful, but the blood transfusion probably would be effective. Even when we substitute Tomlinson's alternative paradigm case, we obtain the same casuistic conclusion, that a court order should be sought. Thus, Tomlinson does not succeed in his attempt to give an example in which alternative paradigms yield different conclusions.

It is not clear that the problem Tomlinson envisages would actually arise, much less arise frequently. However, if alternative sets of paradigms yielded different conclusions, it would raise the issue of whether there is a basis for saying that one set of paradigms is better than the other. This topic would then need to be explored. One possibility is that it would be reasonable to claim that one set of paradigms is preferable — for example, one set might be closer to the case at hand in terms of the morally relevant casuistic factors. In that event, the conclusion indicated by the better set of paradigms would be preferable. If, however, alternative sets of paradigms are equally acceptable, then there are several possibilities. On one hand, they might yield the same conclusion and thereby reinforce each other. On the other hand, if they yielded different conclusions, then the casuist's reply would simply be that casuistry is unable to resolve this particular case. Casuistry makes no claim to resolve all cases. The objection would be serious only if it turned out that frequently there are equally acceptable alternative sets of paradigms that yield different conclusions, but it has not been shown that this occurs.

Another objection by Tomlinson is that casuists cannot articulate the grounds of their decisions. Specifically, he claims that when casuists assert that a given case is close enough to a paradigm case to be decided in the same way as the paradigm, there are no fully articulate grounds for that judgment.[35] This objection overlooks the version of casuistry that I defended in "Justification in Ethics." In that version, one compares the case at hand with two or more paradigm cases. The comparison is based on the extent to which the casuistic factors are present in the various cases. The claim that the case at hand is more like one paradigm than another can be articulated by pointing out the ways in which the casuistic factors in it are more similar to those of one paradigm than to those of another. Casuists do not claim that a clear judgment can always be made. But when it is apparent that the case at hand is more like one paradigm than another, the basis of that claim can be articulated, according to this approach.

Thus, the objections that have been raised do not provide grounds for rejecting the modified casuistic approach.

Summary of the Ethical Framework

This chapter completes the presentation of the ethical framework that will be used in discussing issues in Part 2. The conclusion that this framework is acceptable is stated tentatively for now. A further test will come in Part 2 when we consider the extent to which it is helpful in resolving the issues addressed. The main points of this framework can be summarized as follows.

Procreation is valuable to individuals for various reasons, including the following: (1) it involves participation in the creation of a person; (2) it can be an affirmation of mutual love; (3) it can contribute to sexual intimacy; (4) it can provide a link to future persons; (5) it can result in the experience of pregnancy and childbirth; and (6) it can involve the experience of child rearing. These reasons also suggest that procreating is valuable because it can be important to one's self-identity and self-fulfillment. These reasons for valuing procreation help explain why *freedom* to procreate should be valued and protected.

Moreover, there is a prima facie moral right to noninterference with freedom to procreate, based on respect for persons. Serious interferences with freedom to procreate can adversely affect a person's self-identity and diminish potential for self-fulfillment, and sometimes they violate bodily integrity.

Intentionally to treat individuals in ways likely to result in such harms constitutes a failure to treat them as ends in themselves.

Bearing and raising children is a major undertaking, which can compete with other important life tasks by placing large demands on one's time and resources. For this reason, freedom *not* to procreate is valuable in part because it contributes to self-determination in making major life choices. Self-determination is especially important for women because it is essential for social change toward greater equality for women. In a similar vein, freedom not to procreate is important because it is implied by bodily self-determination, which has special significance for women because they bear the burdens of gestation. Freedom not to procreate is important for self-identity and self-fulfillment because it involves major life decisions. Both freedom to procreate and freedom not to procreate are valuable, ultimately, because of their importance for the self-determination of persons.

Based on consequentialist arguments, normal infants should have a conferred moral standing that is equivalent to normative personhood, including a right to life, even though they are not persons in the descriptive sense. During gestation, the degree of conferred moral standing that embryos and fetuses should have is also based on consequentialist arguments and their degree of similarity with the paradigm of descriptive persons—with normal adult human beings. Morally relevant similarities include the potential to cause self-consciousness, the potential to become self-conscious, viability, sentience, similarity in appearance to the paradigm, birth, and a social role. Fetuses that are relatively advanced in development—sentient fetuses, including those near term—should be regarded as having a conferred right to life, but one that is not quite as strong as that of infants. By contrast, preembryos do not have a right to life, since they lack the potential to become self-conscious, any physical resemblance to descriptive persons, viability, sentience, and a social role. Only a minor degree of moral consideration is justifiable, based on their potential to cause self-consciousness. Embryos also lack a right to life because they have so little similarity to the paradigm. Compared to preembryos, they are slightly more similar to the paradigm because they have the potential to become self-conscious, and the argument for giving them a minor degree of moral consideration because of their symbolic value is perhaps slightly stronger than it is for preembryos. Presentient fetuses have an intermediate moral status. Although a conferred right to life does not seem justifiable, some degree of moral consideration appears warranted, based on their limited similarity to descriptive persons.

In assigning priorities to conflicting ethical values, there is a presumption that the prioritizing should take place in the context of individual cases. Such prioritization is carried out by means of a casuistic approach, and in each case the prioritization must be supported by an argument. Typically, such arguments are based on the extent to which morally relevant casuistic factors are present in the case at hand. However, we should leave open the possibility that for some issues this presumption is overridden by compelling arguments. Such arguments might be based on appeals to consequences or other ethical values having broad social import. Thus, it is conceivable that, for some issues, the same prioritization of conflicting values would be justifiable for all cases in which the issue arises.

PART II

Reproductive and Perinatal Issues

5

Nontraditional Families

Reproductive technology is controversial in part because it makes new types of family arrangements possible. These can be contrasted with the traditional family, in which there are two heterosexual parents, man and woman, who together fulfill the genetic, gestational, and social components of parenting. There are various ways in which families can be unlike this traditional model: the genetic mother and gestational mother might be different persons; the genetic mother and social mother might be different persons; there might be only one social parent; or there might be two social parents of the same sex.

Several main objections have been raised against these nontraditional family arrangements. One is that they are harmful to the children who grow up within them. Another concern is that they are harmful to society because they contribute to the breakdown of the traditional family as a social institution. In addition, it is objected that these arrangements are harmful to women individually and as a group. It is important for us to examine these objections as well as the arguments that support nontraditional families. I propose to examine these pros and cons in the context of several nontraditional family arrangements: artificial insemination for single women, ovum donation for "older" women, and surrogate motherhood.

Artificial Insemination for Single Women

I shall use the term *single women* to refer to unmarried women who either are heterosexual and living without a male partner or are lesbian, whether living with or without a lesbian partner. Several cases will help illustrate the issue of artificial insemination for single women.[1] In the first case, a forty-year-old executive made an appointment with her gynecologist to request artificial insemination by donor.[2] She had never been married, although she currently had a regular sexual partner. Impregnation by this partner would be an alternative, but she did not desire marriage or shared parenthood with this particular man. On her own initiative, she had sought advice from a psychiatrist concerning the impact of single parenthood upon herself and the future child. She brought a letter from the psychiatrist stating that he thought she would be able to cope with the situation satisfactorily. Her family consisted of her parents, a sister, and a brother, none of whom lived close to her. She had discussed with each of them her desire to have a child by artificial insemination, and she stated that they supported her plan. She was in good health and she earned a substantial income. Her parents were wealthy, and she stated that even if she were not working she would be financially secure.

In the second case, a thirty-four-year-old woman who had been divorced for four years requested artificial insemination. She was raising a six-year-old daughter, and she lived with her parents and a brother. She stated that she would consider marrying again, but she currently did not have a romantic involvement with anyone. She wanted to have another child, and she preferred to avoid further delay because she was concerned about the age-related risk of having a child with Down syndrome. She would not choose to abort if the fetus had Down syndrome because she was opposed to abortion. She came from a large family of lower-middle income, and she earned a modest living as a bookkeeper. She had discussed artificial insemination with her parents, and they did not object to her plan. Also, she had discussed with her daughter the possibility of having another child.

Some have argued that donor insemination (DI) for single women is too medicalized, meaning that the assumption often is made that DI must be performed by physicians, whereas it need not be.[3] In support of this view, it is pointed out that some sperm banks will ship frozen sperm directly to single women for self-insemination.[4] Alternatively, a woman can inseminate herself using fresh sperm obtained from a willing male; this is called the "turkey baster" method because that ordinary kitchen implement is all the technology one needs. However, the fact that DI can be performed without the direct assistance of a physician does not diminish the importance of discussing cases like the two presented above. The fact is, single women *do* approach physicians with requests for DI. Moreover, they can have good reasons for doing so: the woman might seek the physician's assurance, for example, that appropriate testing of the sperm for HIV has been performed; or she might have a longstanding relationship with a particular physician and therefore prefer the physician to a sperm bank. My focus will be on the question of how a physician should respond when such requests are made.

DI for single women is an emotional issue for many. Much of the opposition to DI for lesbians is based on widespread disapproval of lesbianism among the general population. Others fiercely defend the right of single women to have children by artificial insemination. The women's rights movement provides a backdrop for this issue. Not many years ago, DI for single women was almost unthinkable, given the traditional attitudes of both men and women concerning the role of women in society. Now women are beginning to be recognized as having equal rights. Feminist authors support DI for single women on the grounds that women should have control over their reproductive lives.[5]

Although requests for DI by single women occur only occasionally, this topic is important in part because it raises a general issue concerning harm to the child that applies not only to DI for single women but to other nontraditional family arrangements arising from new reproductive technologies. Specifically, this is the issue of whether it is accurate to say that it would *harm* a child to bring her into being in circumstances where she would experience disadvantages compared to children in traditional families. This issue hinges partly on the available empirical data concerning whether children raised in nontraditional families actually experience disadvantages. Also — and perhaps more important — its resolution depends on the *logic* of the claim that children are harmed by being brought into being in circumstances in which they experience disadvantages.

We need to explore this issue because one of the main objections to DI for single women is that creating children to be raised in single-mother households is harmful to them. This objection is raised, for example, by I. M. Cosgrove, who states: "How can we ever predict the psychological trauma that might afflict a child conceived in this way? To have collaborated at all in such an event would carry with it an implicit belief, on the part of the doctor, that untold psychological harm will *not,* in all probability, result."[6] A similar view is stated in the Warnock Report, which introduces the topic with the following statement: "To judge from the evidence, many believe that the interests of the child dictate that it should be born into a home where there is a loving, stable, heterosexual relationship and that, therefore, the *deliberate* creation of a child for a woman who is not a partner in such a relationship is morally wrong."[7] The report then states: "We believe that as a general rule it is better for children to be born into a two-parent family, with both father and mother."[8] The implications of this statement emerge later, when the report recommends that DI should be available to infertile couples, thereby excluding single women.[9]

As these statements illustrate, those who object to DI for single women usually are not very specific in stating the supposed harms to children in being conceived and raised by single women. In order to respond to the objections, therefore, we need to consider what specific form they might take. Perhaps the objections are based in part on a concern about the child growing up without a male role model. There has been interest in the effects of the absence of a male role model on a child's development, reflected in a body of literature reporting research on this topic. Much of this literature has focused on the question of whether such children demonstrate appropriate sex-role behavior. A common research technique uses questionnaires to measure degrees of "masculinity" and "femininity." Could it be that those who object to DI for single women are concerned that the boys might grow up to be too feminine?

If this is the concern, then several replies can be made. First, in a review of the literature in question, Elizabeth Herzog and Cecelia E. Sudia found that among studies having acceptable methodology, about half conclude that boys raised in father-absent families are less masculine and about half deny this conclusion.[10] Given these mixed results, Herzog and Sudia concluded that there is no clear correlation between the absence of a father and inappropriate sex-role behavior. Second, many of the studies on sex-role behavior were carried out in the 1950s and 1960s, prior to changes in attitudes brought about by the women's movement, and they reflected stereotypic views concerning the roles of men and women. For example, agreement with the following statements, which were typical items on these questionnaires, would increase a respondent's masculinity score: "I think I would like to drive a racing car" and "At times I feel like picking a fist fight with someone."[11] By contrast, one's femininity score would be increased by agreement with these statements: "A windstorm terrifies me" and "Sometimes I feel that I am about to go to pieces."[12] The underlying views are clear: females should be weak, not daring or aggressive; males should be aggressive, sometimes even belligerent.

Even if boys raised in father-absent families tend to be less masculine according to those questionnaires, it is doubtful that this should be considered an adverse finding. In fact, the entire concern about the sex-role behavior of boys raised by single women seems to be based on those stereotypic views concerning masculinity and femininity. Third, children raised in father-absent families do not completely lack male role models; children learn about sex roles from many sources, including adults in their homes, peer groups, television, movies, and other mass media. Thus, the objection based on sex-role behavior of the offspring is not persuasive.

Similarly, objections to DI for lesbians often are not specific. There have been a few studies addressing the question of whether children raised in lesbian households have an increased tendency to become homosexual. Perhaps the objection is based on a concern that the children will develop such tendencies, in which case two points can be made in reply. First, the objection is not supported by the studies that have been carried out. Richard Green reported a study of twenty-one children of ages five to fourteen raised by lesbian mothers.[13] The subjects were assessed using measures found in previous studies to reflect emerging sexual identity. These included toy and game preferences, peer group composition (which typically is same-sex in grade-school children), clothing preferences, and roles played in fantasy games. For the older children, information was obtained on romantic crushes, erotic fantasies, and sexual behavior. It was found that twenty of the subjects exhibited behavior typical of their sex. The children who reported erotic fantasies or overt sexual behavior were all heterosexually oriented. These results suggest that there is not an increased incidence of homosexual orientation among children raised in lesbian homes, compared to heterosexual households. Confirmation was provided in a study by Martha Kirkpatrick and colleagues, involving a comparison of twenty children raised by lesbian mothers with an equal number raised in father-absent families by heterosexual mothers.[14] The study found no differences in sexual identity between the two groups. Similar results were reported in other studies.[15] Second, the objection is based on the assumption that being homosexual is an adverse outcome. This assumption seems to rest more on prejudice against homosexuals than any objective finding, and it should be rejected.

Perhaps the objection to DI for lesbians is that the children will suffer terribly from the stigma attached to having a lesbian mother. Because of their mothers' lifestyle, they might experience embarrassment, ridicule, difficulties in establishing friendships with other children, and other adverse effects of the negative attitudes of others. In reply, it is undeniable that there would be a stigma, but studies of children raised in lesbian homes suggest that they usually are able to cope satisfactorily with such difficulties. Lesbian mothers realize that their children are stigmatized, and they often encourage open discussion of these matters with their children in order to help them cope.[16] Usually the children understand that the negative views of others are based on prejudice. Rather than being resentful toward their mothers, the children usually believe that society should be faulted for its intolerance.[17] In interviews with twenty-one children raised in lesbian homes, Karen Gail Lewis found that, "almost without exception, the children were proud of their mother for challenging society's rules and for standing up for what she believed."[18]

It might be objected that lesbian relationships are unstable, with breakups causing emotional harm to children caught in the middle. But there is no evidence that the separation rate for lesbian unions is significantly greater than that for heterosexual marriages. According to a study by Marcel Saghir and Eli Robins, having a long-term relationship is usually the intention when a lesbian couple begins living together.[19] As in the case of heterosexual women, lesbians attach importance to the emotional dimensions of a relationship. Sexual gratification in the absence of a shared emotional intimacy and a commitment to each other is generally regarded as unsatisfactory. In contrast to male homosexual relationships, sexual fidelity is a typical characteristic of lesbian couples.[20] Although there is little data available concerning the stability of lesbian relationships, anecdotal evidence indicates that long-term relationships occur.[21] Moreover, it is necessary to keep in mind the current instability of heterosexual relationships, as reflected in high divorce rates. Perhaps it will be objected that the appropriate comparison is between the stability of lesbian relationships and that of heterosexual couples receiving DI. However, there is no data to support the view that there is less stability among lesbian couples than among heterosexual couples receiving DI.

Although the above objections are not persuasive, it should be acknowledged that children raised by single women might experience certain disadvantages in comparison to children raised in two-parent heterosexual households. Besides the disadvantages associated with stigma, there can be financial disadvantages because women generally receive lower salaries than men. The problem of low income is aggravated when there is only one breadwinner, as is the case in many single-mother families. In addition, some offspring might experience psychological discomfort over not knowing who their father is. These disadvantages suggest another way to state the objection. It might simply be claimed that the children are harmed by being born in circumstances where these disadvantages exist. This brings us to the issue I referred to above — whether it is correct to say that children are *harmed* by being brought into being in circumstances where they experience disadvantages compared to other children, given that the only alternative is not to conceive them at all. To explore this issue, we need to consider what is involved in being harmed.

Joel Feinberg has provided detailed discussions of the concept of being harmed, upon which I shall draw.[22] For present purposes, a key point is that persons are harmed only if they are caused to be worse off than they otherwise would have been. As Feinberg puts it, one harms another only if the victim's personal interest is in a worse condition than it would have been had the perpetrator not acted as he did.[23] The claim that DI for single women harms the children who are brought into being, therefore, amounts to saying that the children are *worse off than they would have been if they had not been conceived.* However, do we really want to say this about them?

There are two approaches that can be taken in arguing against this claim. According to one approach, the claim is incoherent because it seems to compare a person's state when she exists to her state when she does not exist; however, when she does not exist, *she* has no state to be compared. However, although the claim in question might initially seem to be incoherent, it is possible to interpret it in a way that avoids this problem. As Feinberg points out, we use expressions like "I would be better off not existing" to convey an idea that in fact is quite intelligible. As he puts it:

> When a miserable adult claims that he would be better off dead, for example, surely he is not making some subtle metaphysical claim implying that there is a realm of being in which even the nonexistent have a place. What he is saying is that he *prefers* to be dead, that is, not to *be* at all. . . . If we speak in the first person, we may be expressing the *wish* (not a desire) that we had never come into existence—Would that I had never been born. When that wish is expressed in terms of being better off not having come into existence, it is to be understood not simply as a wish, but as a claim that the preference implied in the wish is understandable and justifiable, rationally based on the nature of the speaker's present plight. When one party says that another would have been better off had he never been born, he is claiming that the preference for the one state of affairs over the other is a rational preference. Whether true or not, this is an intelligible claim without contradiction or paradox.[24]

Feinberg seems to be correct in arguing that the first approach does not succeed. However, the second approach *is* successful. It states that the claim in question is coherent but false. To see this, let us consider what a life would have to be like in order for us reasonably to say that it is worse for the person living it than nonexistence. To use Feinberg's terminology, what would it have to be like in order for the preference for nonexistence to be justifiable? I would like to suggest that a life would have to be so filled with pain or other forms of suffering that these negative experiences greatly overshadowed any pleasurable or other positive experiences the individual might have. If an infant were born with a painful, debilitating, and fatal genetic disease, for example, we could reasonably make such a statement. However, the gulf between such a life and that of a child raised in a single-parent family is exceedingly broad. Children of single women do not have lives filled with pain and suffering. On the contrary, by being brought into existence they are given the opportunity to experience the joys of living and to make of their lives what they will. Admittedly, they will experience pains as well as pleasures, as all of us do. However, the disadvantages experienced by children raised by single women — lower incomes and difficulties associated with stigma — are not severe enough to warrant a judgment that their lives are worse than nonexistence. Thus, the objection that DI for single women harms the children is simply confused and mistaken.

I have applied the usual concept of harm to situations involving bringing a child into being. However, there is an objection that we should consider. It might be claimed that applying this concept of harm to this type of situation leads to implausible conclusions. In particular, it seems to imply that there is nothing wrong with knowingly creating a child who will suffer disadvantages — even *serious* ones — as long as those disadvantages are not so severe that the life will be worse than nonexistence. Consider an example in which the single woman who requests artificial insemination is an alcoholic and has not been rehabilitated. Suppose that a physician knows about the alcoholism but performs DI, and the child later has fetal alcohol syndrome, with associated facial stigmata and mental retardation.[25] It seems wrong for a physician to carry out DI for a woman who is an unreformed alcoholic. According to the usual concept of harm, however, the child in this example is not harmed by the act of performing DI, given that the child's life is better than nonexistence. If we cannot say that the child is harmed, then how can we account for our view that performing the DI is unethical? Perhaps we should develop a new definition of harm to apply to this type of situation.

In reply, we can account for DI being unethical in such a case without inventing a new concept of harm. Although the child is not harmed by the DI, we can say that he is *wronged*. In particular, we can say that a certain *right* of the child is violated. Others have suggested that there might be a type of *birthright*, according to which people have a right to be born free of serious impediments to their well-being.[26] It is important to be clear about the nature of this right. It is *not* a "right to be born" but rather a right possessed by all who *are* born and have the status of normative personhood. It also is not what one might call a "right against nature." A child born with serious handicaps, through the fault of no one, cannot claim that the right in question is violated. Rather, like all rights, this one is a type of moral relationship between individuals. The right would only be violated if someone intentionally or negligently caused a child to be born with the requisite impediments. I would like to suggest that we can account for the wrongness of DI in the alcoholism example by positing such a birthright, a right that one's circumstances of birth be free of impediments that would seriously impair one's ability to develop in a healthy manner and to realize a normal potential. Intentionally or negligently to bring into being a child who faces such severe impediments is to violate that right, which I shall refer to as a right to a decent minimum opportunity for development. The impediments imposed on the child with fetal alcohol syndrome are not so severe that we could reasonably say that her life is worse than nonexistence, but they are severe enough to impair seriously her ability to develop.

One can defend the claim that there is such a right, using the account of rights I presented in Chapter 1. I argued that a person has a *right* to be free of an interference if that interference constitutes treating the person as a mere means and not as an end in herself. Performing DI when there is a significant chance that the child will have serious impairments threatens the child's ability to pursue her own ends. If the impairments materialize, then they will constitute an interference with the child's capacity to do things; there will be a reduction in her ability to pursue her well-being and a diminution in her range of feasible options for choosing plans for her life. Moreover, we can say that the DI fails to treat the child as an end in herself because it is reasonably foreseeable that there is a significant likelihood of a major reduction in her ability to select and pursue ends of her own choosing.

An objection can be made against using the concept "being wronged" to describe what is unethical about the DI in the above example. Feinberg raises the objection when considering congenital handicaps that are serious, but not serious enough to warrant the claim that the child's life is worse than nonexistence. Feinberg's hypothetical example involves a woman who knows that if she conceives at a certain time, then her child will have a defect—a withered arm. Nevertheless, whether through intentional perversity or reckless impulsiveness, she conceives at the dangerous time and the child has the defect.[27] According to Feinberg, the mother did not *wrong* the child by causing him to come into being in a handicapped condition. Feinberg argues that if the child were to claim that he was wronged, it would commit him to the judgment that her duty to him had been to refrain from doing what she did; but if she had refrained, it would have led to his never having been born, an even worse result from his point of view.[28] Thus, according to Feinberg, the child cannot reasonably claim that his mother *should* have acted otherwise, given that his life with a withered arm is preferable to nonexistence. If he cannot make this claim, then he has no genuine grievance against her and cannot claim that she wronged him.

I believe that Feinberg's argument is mistaken. Perhaps we can see this more clearly if we consider a similar type of situation. Instead of actions that cause a person to come into being, let us consider acts that cause an existing person to continue to live — that is, *life-saving acts*. Both types of actions have the result that a person exists who otherwise would not be in existence. Consider a patient who has suffered substantial bleeding because of a ruptured gastric ulcer. Suppose that blood transfusions are necessary to save her life, but she refuses transfusions for religious reasons and is considered to be mentally competent. Imagine that the physician provides the transfusions anyway, with the result that the patient's life is saved. Let us suppose, also, that the patient later acknowledges that she is better off having been kept alive. According to Feinberg's reasoning, the patient cannot reasonably claim that the physician should have refrained from treating, given that her continued life is preferable to nonexistence. If she cannot make this claim, then she cannot claim that the physician wronged her.

However, this conclusion is incorrect. Clearly, the patient can validly claim that she was wronged; her right to informed consent and right to self-determination were violated. The beneficial outcome of the physician's action does not alter the fact that these rights were infringed. If a good outcome removed all wrongness of the act, that would mean that paternalism, when successfully carried out, is always ethically justifiable. This would be inconsistent with our view that competent patients have a right to refuse life-saving treatment. Similarly, the fact that the child with the withered arm has a life that is better than nonexistence does not mean that the child was not wronged. More generally, a child who is intentionally or negligently brought into being in circumstances where there is not a decent minimum opportunity for development is wronged, even if her life is better than nonexistence, just as a competent patient who is forced to receive life-saving treatment is wronged, even though her subsequent life is better than nonexistence.

Given the idea that there is a right to a decent minimum opportunity for development, some might claim that artificial insemination for single women usually, if not always, violates this right because of the disadvantages the children experience. However, it seems implausible that these disadvantages are severe enough to constitute a violation of the right in question. If this is a violation, then it seems to follow that the right is violated for all children intentionally conceived by heterosexual couples who have a low income. Similarly, we would have to say that the right is violated whenever it is likely that the child will suffer from stigma, a problem that racial and ethnic minorities often face. However, these conclusions do not seem reasonable. Of course, if there is a right to a decent minimum opportunity for development, then the question arises concerning how serious the impediments must be in order for the right to be violated. No doubt, there is room for disagreement concerning this question, and a sharp line probably cannot be drawn. Nevertheless, a basic concept can be articulated: the impediments must be severe, not minor. As examples, I would suggest that a withered arm or fetal alcohol syndrome are severe enough, but being born into a family with an income that is merely below-average (as distinct from being born into abject poverty) is not.

The above discussion gives us a new perspective on the empirical research concerning children raised by single women. Many who have defended DI for single women have used that body of research to argue that supposed adverse effects—increased femininity among boys, increased tendency toward homosexuality, and so forth—do not occur. I used that approach myself in the above discussion and earlier article.[29] However, in discussing the logical flaw in the objection that DI for single women harms the children who would be created, we have seen that even if there are adverse effects of being raised in father-absent homes, they do not constitute a reason against performing DI for single women unless they severely interfere with a child's opportunity for development. Thus, the burden of defending DI for single women does not rest as heavily on the results of empirical research as some might think. It is not necessary to show that there are *no* disadvantages associated with being raised in father-absent homes, only that there are no *severe* disadvantages.[30]

A persistent opponent of DI for single women might fall back to another position: that such DI is wrong because it fails to satisfy some ideal of child rearing. On this view, any disadvantages associated with being raised by single mothers, while not severe enough to constitute harms or wrongs, constitute a failure to meet some specified ideal. But the view that procreation is wrong unless the child would be raised in some set of ideal conditions is unsupportable. In the world around us, many children are born into conditions that are less than ideal, involving hardships, unstable social conditions, or physical dangers (as in some violence-prone neighborhoods or countries). However, it would not be reasonable to say that people in such settings should not have children, unless perhaps the adverse conditions were extreme. Moreover, the objection assumes that a single-mother home could not meet a reasonable ideal. However, if the child is loved, nurtured, guided, and respected as a person, why should that not count as a valid ideal?

Another objection is based on concern for the well-being of society. DI for single women, it is claimed, will contribute to a breakdown of the traditional pattern of two-parent heterosexual families, with a resulting change in social values characterized by less importance given to traditional family life. In reply, it is reasonable to believe that most people will continue to choose heterosexual marriage as the basis of family life. Thus, it is unlikely that DI for single women will significantly contribute to a breakdown of the sort in question. Moreover, the important values associated with family—such as love, caring, and fidelity — can exist in nontraditional families as well as traditional ones. It is doubtful, therefore, that the existence of nontraditional families undermines these important values.

In addition, there is a positive argument supporting DI for single women — carrying out such requests promotes freedom to procreate and the happiness of women. According to a recent survey, a majority of lesbian women desire to have children.[31] Similarly, it is not unusual for single heterosexual women to want children. In Chapter 1, we considered a number of reasons why procreating can be meaningful to persons. Some of them are reasons that can be important to single women: to participate in the creation of a person; to have a link with future persons; and to experience pregnancy, childbirth, and child rearing.

If, as I have argued, it is sometimes ethically justifiable for physicians to carry out requests for DI by single women, then under what circumstances would it *not* be justifiable? It seems that one type of circumstance would be cases where pregnancy involves high risks for the woman. Examples might include women with advanced diabetes or heart disease. It can be argued that there is a significant chance that the physician would violate the principle "do no harm" in providing DI in such cases. Another type of situation would be cases where there is a substantial risk of serious handicaps for the child. If the potential handicaps are severe enough to deprive the child of a decent minimum opportunity for development, then the physician should not proceed if there is a high enough probability that the handicaps will materialize. An example would be a woman who is alcoholic, as discussed above. Another example would be a woman who is HIV-positive, where there is approximately a 20 to 30 percent chance of transmitting HIV infection to the fetus.[32] It would be wrong for the physician to provide DI to single women with these medical problems. These considerations indicate that the physician should obtain a medical history and perform a physical examination of the single woman before carrying out DI. This implies that the physician's decision concerning whether to carry out the woman's request should be made on a case-by-case basis, in accordance with the modified casuistic approach for which I argued in Chapter 4.

When physicians carry out such requests, part of their role is to offer counseling to help the woman make an informed and voluntary decision. If there are any medical risks to the woman or potential child, these should be discussed. Being informed includes being aware of potential problems that can arise for single women having children, and counseling can address the possible emotional, psychological, and legal difficulties. It can also address the desirability of a support system, such as family or friends who would be available to help care for the child in the event of maternal illness or financial difficulties. Many single women seeking DI have thought through the decision carefully before approaching a physician,[33] and some may need little counseling.

The view I am defending can be applied to the two case examples presented above. In the case of the forty-year-old executive, the patient was counseled concerning the increased risk of congenital anomalies due to her age. She replied that she would want an amniocentesis and would consider abortion if there were a major genetic defect. She stated that her family was available as a support system if she ever were to become ill. After discussing DI with the patient, the physician was convinced that she had thought carefully about the various ramifications of her decision. All things considered, this was a case in which it was ethically permissible for the physician to carry out the request. In the case of the thirty-four-year-old woman, if the DI were carried out relatively soon, she would not have a significant risk of producing a child with a genetic disease. There was a large, close family that was capable of providing a support system for the woman and her children. She was counseled concerning the various aspects of the situation. In this case, as in the first, carrying out the request would be ethically permissible.

My arguments support the view that it is ethically permissible for physicians to carry out DI for single women, but not that it is obligatory to do so. A physician who conscientiously objects to fulfilling a single woman's request for DI has a right to refuse.

Although I have focused on physician ethics, another important question is whether it is ethical for the single woman to undergo DI. The above discussion helps us answer this question. In Chapter 3, I stated that procreators have an obligation to act beneficently toward their offspring. The above discussion suggests one of the implications of this: there is an obligation to avoid procreating when there is a significant likelihood that the child's right to a decent minimum opportunity for development would be violated. We can conclude that it is ethically permissible for single women to undergo DI unless doing so would violate this obligation. This implies, for example, that it would be wrong for single women who are alcoholic or HIV-positive to undergo DI, given a lack of methods to detect prenatally or cure the fatal conditions.

Ovum Donation for Older Women

Ovum donation is a technique for helping infertile couples that was introduced relatively recently. It involves giving superovulation drugs to a donor, followed by oocyte recovery. A common recovery method involves insertion of a needle transvaginally and aspiration of oocytes, using ultrasound for guidance. The oocytes then are combined with the recipient's husband's sperm in vitro. Depending on how many preembryos are formed, from one to five preembryos are transferred to the recipient's uterus. Typically, the donor is a volunteer who undergoes oocyte recovery solely for the purpose of donation. She can be anonymous, or in some cases might be a friend or relative of the recipient. Anonymous donors usually are matched with recipients, at least to some extent, according to physical characteristics. The process is a carefully planned one involving timed administration of estradiol and progesterone to the recipient in order to synchronize the menstrual cycles of donor and recipient and prepare the recipient's endometrium to receive the preembryos. Ovum donation originally was introduced to address several types of medical problems: infertility due to premature ovarian failure, a condition in which the ovaries no longer produce oocytes; for women whose ovaries have been surgically removed as part of treatment for conditions such as infection or endometriosis, but who have a retained uterus; and to avoid transmission of genetic disease. More recently, ovum donation has been used for infertile women over forty years of age when in vitro fertilization (IVF) with their own oocytes has been unsuccessful and there is no explanation for infertility other than age. It has been discovered that success rates improve dramatically when ova from younger donors are used, rather than the over-forty patient's own ova.[34] The realization that ovum donation can be effective for woman over forty paved the way for its use by postmenopausal women.

Rosanna Dalla Corte, a sixty-two-year-old Italian woman who used ovum donation, made the headlines when she gave birth to a seven-pound boy in June 1994.[35] She and her sixty-five-year-old husband had lost their only child, Ricardo, when he had died three years earlier in a motorcycle accident at age eighteen. They wanted another child and tried to adopt but were unable to do so under Italian law because they were too old. Mrs. Dalla Corte became a patient of Dr. Severino Antinori, a Rome gynecologist well known in Europe for treating older women who can no longer conceive naturally. After becoming pregnant using ovum donation, she stated, "I have suffered much, so why shouldn't I now deserve the joy of raising a new baby? . . . It is a very big responsibility, but I am nevertheless sure that I will have much love to give it, an infinite love."[36] The new baby also was named Ricardo. This case occurred soon after another of Antinori's patients, a fifty-nine-year-old British woman, received world-wide media attention. The British patient, whose name was not disclosed, gave birth to twins following oocyte donation.[37]

In response to these cases, there were many comments, positive and negative. In France, Health Minister Philippe Douste-Blazy stated, "I think it is absolutely shocking that a child can be eighteen when his mother is eighty. It is totally undeserved." He announced that the French government would introduce legislation to ban ovum donation for postmenopausal women.[38] The British secretary of state for health, Virginia Bottomly, asserted that "women do not have a right to have children." She declared that the British government would not permit ovum donation for postmenopausal women.[39] As these comments suggest, ovum donation for older women raises issues concerning procreative freedom. Specifically, at least two ethical questions can be distinguished: Is ovum donation for older women ethically justifiable, and should ovum donation for older women be legally banned?

Before addressing these issues, we need to ask what is meant by the vague term "older" women. Douste-Blazy and Bottomly referred to postmenopausal women, and for the purposes of this discussion I shall assume that objections to ovum donation for older women are directed primarily at postmenopausal women. This group, therefore, will be the main focus of attention.

IS OVUM DONATION FOR OLDER WOMEN ETHICALLY JUSTIFIABLE?

At least three objections have been put forward against ovum donation for older women. First, it has been argued that it should not be permitted because pregnancy and childbirth involve increased risks to the older woman. This objection is based on a body of literature dealing with the effects of advanced maternal age on pregnancy. Interestingly, in most of this literature, advanced maternal age is defined as thirty-five or older. Although there are conflicting reports within this body of literature, overall it supports the view that advanced maternal age is associated with an increased incidence of complications of pregnancy, including hypertension, diabetes, *placenta previa, abruptio placentae,* and cesarean section.[40] Within this body of literature, little data is available concerning pregnancy complications for patients over the age of forty-five. Thus, the extent of risk for women over forty-five is unknown.

In reply to this objection, several points can be made. First, the maternal risks can be reduced by screening potential ovum recipients for health problems, including cardiovascular problems and diabetes, and by closely monitoring the mother's health status during pregnancy.[41] Second, patients should be allowed to assume at least some degree of risk, based on their own values, provided they are mentally competent and adequately informed of the risks. In this context, being adequately informed includes being told that the level of risk is unknown for older women free of preconception health problems.

A second objection is that caring for children is more difficult for older people. Raising children is an energy-consuming task, and some older persons might regret becoming parents late in life because they do not have the stamina required. However, it can be pointed out that many children have been raised

by grandparents. This provides evidence that older people are capable of fulfilling parental roles. Also, we allow older persons to undertake other arduous
endeavors, so why should we not allow them to undertake child rearing?[42] To
prevent ovum donation for older women because of the objection in question
would be unjustifiably paternalistic.

Third, it can be objected that there is an increased likelihood that one or
both parents would die before the child is raised and, therefore, there is a risk
of harm to the child due to parental death. This objection makes the same
mistake concerning the concept of harm that I discussed above in connection
with DI for single women. If it were not for the ovum donation in question, the
child would not exist. The objection therefore amounts to saying that the
children whose parents die are worse off than they would have been if they had
not been conceived. However, it seems unreasonable to make this claim. Having a parent die is not equivalent to having a life so filled with pain and
suffering that these negative experiences outweigh any positive experiences
that might occur. Although there is psychological trauma associated with
parental death, one would expect that the children's lives would contain many
positive experiences, as well, and that they would regard their lives as worth
living.

Perhaps it will be objected that if parental death occurs during the child's
tender years, then the right to a decent minimum opportunity for development
will be violated. It must be acknowledged that parental death can be a setback
to a child's development. The question is whether it typically would be such a
serious setback that it would constitute a violation of the right in question. We
would need to consider both the severity and the probability of the setback. If
only one parent dies, then the surviving parent will raise the child. Having only
one parent, however, does not seem to constitute such a severe obstacle to
development that we would say that the right is violated. If both parents die,
the setback will be more severe. The child will be raised by others — either
relatives or foster or adoptive parents, or in an institution. Even if loving care
were provided, the child's life likely would be significantly disrupted. The
likelihood of both parents dying, however, can be assessed by considering life
expectancies. If we assume that the couple is sixty when the child is born, then
the life expectancy would be another twenty-three years for the woman and
nineteen years for the man.[43] Thus, *on average,* the child would be a young
adult before both parents died. This suggests that it is likely that there would
not be a severe setback. These considerations support the view that ovum
donation for older women does not involve a significant risk of violating the
right in question.

In addition, positive arguments can be given supporting ovum donation for older women, based on the reasons for valuing freedom to procreate discussed in Chapter 1. To begin, it is worth noting that all of those reasons can be considered important to "older" persons. A relatively older couple might value procreation for any of the following reasons: it involves participation in the creation of a person; it can affirm mutual love; it can contribute to sexual intimacy; it provides a link to future persons; it involves experiences of pregnancy and childbirth; and it can lead to experiences associated with child rearing.

These are reasons why having *genetic* offspring can be important to persons. Let us consider the extent to which these reasons have implications for ovum donation, where the recipient will be the gestational but not the genetic mother. First, the recipient's male partner *will* be the genetic father of any children who are brought into being by the oocyte donation, and a number of the reasons identified could be considered important to him. He would participate in the creation of a person, have a genetic link to future persons, and expect to have experiences of child rearing. Also, although his partner is not the genetic mother, he might well regard their mutual desire for her to gestate his genetic offspring to be an affirmation of each other's love. Second, several of the identified reasons would be relevant to the oocyte recipient. Through her gestational role, she would participate in the creation of a person. She, too, might regard her procreative contribution as an affirmation of mutual love. Although she would not have a genetic link, she would have a familial link to future persons, based on her role as gestational and social mother. In addition, she could expect to have experiences of pregnancy, childbirth, and child rearing. The only reason listed in Chapter 1 that is not relevant either to the oocyte recipient or to her male partner is procreation's contribution to sexual intimacy, since ovum donation does not involve sexual intercourse. All things considered, ovum donation for older women can satisfy reasonable desires, the fulfillment of which promotes the well-being and autonomy of the individuals involved. These considerations support the view that it is ethically justifiable for physicians to provide ovum donation to older women, at least in some cases.

However, there might be several types of situations in which it is *not* ethically justifiable for physicians to carry out requests for ovum donation by older women. One type would be that in which there are significant risks to the health or life of the woman. Examples would include women with diabetes or heart disease; also, in the future we might learn that above a certain age there are high risks of some sort to pregnant women. Physicians have an important obligation to avoid causing harm to their patients. If the maternal risks are high enough, this obligation suggests that it would be ethically preferable to refuse the patient's request. Another type of case would be that in which there is a significant risk of major handicaps for the child. Perhaps in the future we shall learn that above a certain maternal age there are significant nongenetic risks of birth injury to the child.[44] However, the handicaps would have to be severe enough that the child's right to a minimum decent opportunity for development would be violated. A third type of situation would be that in which there are serious impairments to the voluntary informed consent of the woman. An example might be a case in which the woman seems ambivalent about becoming pregnant and is being pressured by her husband to have a child. These considerations imply, once again, that the physician's decisions should be made on a case-by-case basis, in accordance with the modified casuistic approach.

If it is ethically justifiable for a physician to provide ovum donation for an older woman in a given case, would it nevertheless be ethical for the physician to refuse to participate? I suggest that the answer is yes. Because we are dealing with a controversial ethical issue, the principle of conscientious objection seems applicable. Some physicians might conscientiously object, for example, because of concern that their actions might violate the principle to do no harm, given that the risks are unknown.

SHOULD THERE BE A LEGAL BAN?

Although some have expressed the view that ovum donation for older women should be legally forbidden, there are ethical and legal arguments against such a ban. Let us begin with an ethical argument. We have seen that there are reasons for valuing freedom to procreate and that these reasons are applicable to relatively older couples. I argued that these reasons provide the basis of procreative rights, including a prima facie right to noninterference with freedom to procreate. Laws forbidding ovum donation for older women would constitute an interference with this right and would be unjustifiable unless there are countervailing reasons that outweigh the right. However, we have examined the main objections to ovum donation for older women and found them to be unpersuasive. Thus, they do not have sufficient merit to override freedom to procreate.

The legal argument against a ban in the United States also is based on ethical considerations but employs concepts of constitutional law. In a long line of cases, the U.S. Supreme Court has maintained that freedom *not to procreate* deserves protection as a fundamental right.[45] Although the Court has never explicitly stated that freedom *to procreate* has fundamental-right status, several considerations support the view that it should have this status. First, in several cases the Court has strongly implied that freedom to procreate is a fundamental right. In *Skinner v. Oklahoma*, the Court made the following statement concerning Oklahoma's sterilization law: "We are dealing here with legislation which involves one of the basic civil rights of man. Marriage and procreation are fundamental to the very existence and survival of the race."[46] In *Loving v. Virginia*, the Court struck down Virginia's law against interracial marriages, thereby protecting a freedom closely related to freedom to procreate — freedom to choose one's spouse.[47] Similarly, in *Stanley v. Illinois* the Court overturned an Illinois law that authorized the removal of children from the custody of the unmarried genetic father upon the death of the mother.[48] In doing so, the Court protected something that is part of the right to procreate — the right of natural parents to raise their children. In its decision, the Court stated: "The private interest here, that of a man in the children he has sired and raised, undeniably warrants deference and, absent a powerful countervailing interest, protection. . . . The Court has frequently emphasized the importance of the family. The rights to conceive and to raise one's children have been deemed 'essential,' Meyer v. Nebraska, . . . 'basic civil rights of man,' Skinner v. Oklahoma, . . . and '[r]ights far more precious . . . than property rights,' May v. Anderson."[49] Second, if freedom not to procreate deserves protection as a fundamental right, then it would be unreasonable to deny such protection to freedom to procreate. Both are important freedoms that have a crucial bearing on self-identity and self-determination. There is no reason to think that freedom to procreate is significantly less important than freedom not to procreate.

If freedom to procreate should be recognized as a fundamental right, then laws infringing it should receive "strict scrutiny" by the Court. This means that a compelling state interest would be needed to override this freedom. However, based on the above examination of ethical objections to ovum donation for older women, it appears that compelling reasons for interference do not exist.

Surrogate Motherhood

There are three kinds of reasons why a couple might wish to procreate in collaboration with a surrogate mother. The most common reason is that the couple is infertile and there is no other avenue for them to have a child who is genetically related to at least one of them. This situation might arise because the woman's uterus has been surgically removed or attempts at in vitro fertilization (IVF) have been unsuccessful.[50] A second reason is that pregnancy might pose significant health risks to the woman, as in cases of heart disease or advanced diabetes. The third possible reason is to avoid inconvenience for the couple. An example might involve a woman who wants a child but does not want pregnancy to interfere with her career. This third reason is not likely to occur with any significant frequency in the near future; few women seem to have this combination of motivations, and the high cost of IVF will be an additional barrier.

Few issues in reproductive ethics have received greater attention than surrogate motherhood. Innumerable articles have been written and many different views have been expressed. Since the highly publicized case of "Baby M" in 1988,[51] many states in the U. S. have passed laws concerning surrogate motherhood, and these laws reflect a diversity of approaches to the question of what social policies we should have.

Much of the debate concerning social policy revolves around three main questions. First, should surrogate motherhood be legally permitted? Discussions of this topic usually make a distinction between *commercial* surrogacy, which typically involves monetary payments to the surrogate mother and to an agent who sets up the surrogacy arrangement, and *noncommercial* surrogacy, which usually is privately arranged and involves a surrogate who is a friend or relative of the infertile couple.[52] Second, if surrogacy is legally permitted, should surrogacy contracts be legally enforceable? Third, if surrogacy is permitted, should it be regulated and, if so, what regulations should there be? Should the regulations attempt to discourage surrogacy?

Depending on how one answers these questions, a number of different views are possible. However, most of these can be grouped under five main views. To explore the question of what our social policies should be, I shall try to point out the pros and cons of these main views.

1. *Commercial and noncommercial surrogacy should be legally prohibited.* This represents one pole of the spectrum of views, being the most restrictive. It is illustrated by Arizona's surrogacy law, passed in 1989, which states: "No person may enter into, induce, arrange, procure, or otherwise assist in the formation of a surrogate parentage contract."[53] For the purposes of this statute, "contract" is defined to include surrogacy "agreements" and "arrangements." Thus, the prohibition covers commercial and noncommercial surrogacy. Another illustration is the view stated in the Catholic church's *Donum Vitae,* which opposes all forms of collaborative reproduction.[54]

2. *Commercial surrogacy should be legally prohibited, and noncommercial surrogacy should be permitted but discouraged.* An example of this view is Utah's surrogacy law, enacted in 1989, which makes it a misdemeanor to be a party to a commercial surrogacy contract.[55] The statute discourages noncommercial surrogacy by creating obstacles to the infertile couple becoming the legal parents of the child. It does this by making such arrange-

ments legally unenforceable, declaring the surrogate mother to be the mother of the child for all legal purposes, declaring her husband (if she is married) to be the legal father, and stipulating that decisions concerning custody will be based solely on the best interests of the child.[56]

3. *Commercial surrogacy should be legally prohibited, and noncommercial surrogacy should be regulated without discouraging it.* This view is illustrated by the New Hampshire surrogacy law, passed in 1990.[57] According to this statute, receiving fees to arrange surrogate motherhood contracts is a misdemeanor. Noncommercial surrogacy contracts are legal if and only if they are judicially preauthorized by a probate court. The regulation of surrogacy involves a number of requirements, including psychological counseling of all parties, genetic counseling if the surrogate is thirty-five years of age or older, and restriction of surrogate motherhood to women with at least one previous pregnancy and viable delivery.[58]

4. *Commercial and noncommercial surrogacy should be legally permitted, and both should be regulated without discouraging them.* This view is embodied in the Model Surrogacy Act of the Section of Family Law of the American Bar Association.[59] This model act proposes a number of regulations, including required medical and psychological examinations and counseling, required term life insurance for the surrogate, and a statement of remedies that will be legally recognized if there is a breach of contract. In addition, a number of authors have advocated this fourth viewpoint.[60]

5. *Commercial and noncommercial surrogacy should be legally permitted; surrogacy contracts should be enforceable, and no special restrictions should be placed on them.* This represents the opposite pole, being the least restrictive option.

To consider the pros and cons of these views, let us begin with the two extreme positions. A difficulty with the first view is that it overlooks the reasons for valuing freedom to procreate that were identified in Chapter 1. In that chapter, I argued that interferences with this freedom violate a moral right to reproduce. Similarly, laws that forbid surrogacy arrangements infringe upon this right. In order for such infringements to be justifiable, there must be countervailing moral reasons of sufficient weight to override the right to reproduce. However, there do not appear to be countervailing reasons of sufficient weight to support the first view, particularly in light of the fact that this view forbids noncommercial surrogacy. Certain types of noncommercial surrogacy arrangements seem to be examples of ethically justifiable surrogacy. I have in mind cases in which a woman volunteers to be a surrogate mother for her infertile sister. The cases of this type that have been reported seem generally to have a favorable outcome for all the parties involved. Because the first view would unjustifiably outlaw such arrangements, it should be rejected.

The difficulty with view 5 is that it fails to deal with the problems that sometimes arise in surrogacy cases. One of the most widely recognized problems is that some surrogate mothers become so psychologically attached to the child that they change their mind about giving it up. Highly publicized cases in which this happened involved Mary Beth Whitehead[61] and Anna Johnson.[62] It seems unwise to permit surrogacy without measures that attempt to reduce the incidence of this problem. Such measures might involve preconception counseling and screening of potential surrogate mothers in an attempt to identify, if possible, those who seem to be at especially high risk of later deciding to keep the child. However, if there is no regulation, then this and other safeguards might not be used. Another type of problem can arise if the child is born with handicaps. The commissioning couple might refuse to accept the child, as happened in a case involving an infant with microcephaly.[63] If the child has handicaps through no fault of the surrogate, then the commissioning couple should not be allowed to refuse to take the child from her. For these reasons, view 5 is unsatisfactory. Views 1 and 5 seem to be examples of an approach to the prioritization of values that I argued against in Chapter 4: the approach in which prioritization is always made in the context of a certain *type* of case, as opposed to individual cases.

To assess the remaining views, let us consider whether commercial surrogacy should be prohibited. Several main arguments have been put forward in favor of forbidding it, and we need to consider whether they are sufficiently weighty to override the right to reproduce. First, it is claimed that surrogate motherhood is psychologically harmful to the children. One specific concern is that harm might occur if the children learn that they were relinquished by the biological mother. This argument makes the same mistake concerning the concept of harm that I discussed in regard to DI for single women and ovum donation for older women, and it should be rejected.

Second, it is argued that commercial surrogacy is degrading to women because it treats a woman's ability to gestate like any other service in the marketplace. This argument and the remaining arguments against commercial surrogacy that I shall discuss are often put forward by feminist writers,[64] although they are asserted by nonfeminists as well. However, even among feminists there is disagreement concerning the merits of these arguments.[65] One version of this argument is put forward by Elizabeth S. Anderson, who attempts to explain why she considers it demeaning to women to treat gestation as a service.[66] She claims that it is natural for a woman to bond with her fetus, but surrogacy requires the woman to repress whatever parental love she feels. Thus, surrogacy demeans her because it is not sensitive to her emotional relationship to the child. But, as Debra Satz points out, not all women bond with their fetuses; some women have abortions.[67] Even among women who do not abort, not all bond to their children. Also, the objection is tied to traditional attitudes about pregnancy and mothering. It seems to assume a norm in which all pregnant women *should* develop a strong attachment to the fetus. However, the new reproductive technologies make new roles possible. Now a woman can choose a partial role in procreation — for example, gestating but not raising, or begetting and gestating but not raising. These new roles invite new attitudes and expectations concerning, among other things, the woman's emotional attachment to the child. The emotional dimensions of pregnancy as a surrogate mother need not be the same as the emotional aspects of a pregnancy in which the woman intends from the beginning to raise the child; this has been demonstrated by many surrogate mothers who have gestated without developing a conviction that they must keep the child. Why assume that we should cling to the traditional roles? Moreover, it is not necessarily degrading to be in a position in which one is called upon to repress one's feelings toward others. Consider, for example, doctors and nurses who constantly care for dying patients. It is common for them to distance themselves emotionally, to some extent, in order to preserve their own psychological health. Should we say, therefore, that it is degrading to be a doctor or nurse?

Rather than say that surrogacy is degrading to women, it would perhaps be more accurate to say that it carries a risk of psychological harm to some women. This claim constitutes a third argument against commercial surrogacy. However, from the fact that some women are at risk, it does not necessarily follow that surrogacy should be forbidden. We should consider whether these risks outweigh the considerations in support of commercial surrogacy. A main argument in support of it is that it promotes the well-being and reproductive liberty of some infertile couples. For some, it brings an end to the anguish of infertility. Another argument is that some surrogate mothers find this type of participation in procreation to be highly meaningful. These positive aspects of surrogacy should not be disregarded. If the risks of psychological harm to surrogate mothers can be kept relatively low by careful screening and counseling of potential surrogates, then it is not obvious that those risks should outweigh the positive aspects of commercial surrogacy.

Fourth, it is argued that commercial surrogacy is demeaning to the child because it treats the child as a commodity and, in fact, is a form of baby selling. In reply, several points can be made. First, the fact that money changes hands does not necessarily transform surrogacy into baby selling. Money paid to a surrogate can be — and should be — regarded as compensation for the time, discomforts, and risks she undergoes in providing her biological services in an attempt to create a baby. It might be objected that some surrogacy contracts provide for payment only if there is a live birth, and in such cases the fee seems to be payment for a baby rather than for the woman's time and risks. Laura Purdy responds to this objection by arguing that payment should not be contingent upon a live birth.[68] It is unfair to the surrogate mother to make the payment contingent in this way. If she provides the biological services agreed upon, then she should be paid; childbearing never carries with it the guarantee of a live birth. If payment is not contingent on a live birth, then it is difficult to maintain that surrogacy is baby selling. Second, there is an important moral difference between entering an agreement to sell a baby who already exists and entering a commercial surrogacy agreement. Selling existing babies clearly amounts to treating them as mere means and not as ends in themselves. From the seller's point of view, the baby is a means to financial gain. In surrogacy, however, the surrogate mother does not treat the fetus or child as a mere means. During gestation, typically, she promotes the interests of the fetus by obtaining prenatal care, eating nutritious meals, and avoiding behavior that would seriously jeopardize the fetus's health. This is treating the future child as an end in himself. Moreover, without the surrogate mother, the child would never exist, never have ends of his own. It is the surrogacy, in fact, that causes the coming into being of an end in himself, the child. Thus, the surrogate mother not only *treats* the child as an end in himself, she helps *create* the child as an end in himself.

A fifth argument is that commercial surrogacy diminishes the autonomy of women.[69] Those who put forward this argument point out that surrogacy contracts contain provisions that restrict the liberty of the surrogate. For example, typically she is required to obtain prenatal care and avoid smoking, alcohol, and drugs, except for medicines prescribed by her physician. She also agrees to undergo amniocentesis and abort if there is a fetal malformation and abortion is desired by the father. However, the restrictions that aim to promote the well being of the fetus, such as avoiding smoking and obtaining prenatal care, are no more than is morally required of any pregnant woman.[70] It does not seem morally objectionable for the surrogate to agree to restrict her behavior in these ways. Other sorts of restrictions — such as requirements to undergo amniocentesis and abort if requested — are indeed problematic. If a woman changes her mind and prefers not to undergo these procedures, her wishes should prevail; she has the right to make decisions concerning medical procedures performed on her body. To force her to undergo such procedures would be an unjustifiable infringement of her autonomy, and to include such requirements in the contract would be coercive. However, these infringements of autonomy can be prevented by not allowing surrogacy contracts to contain such provisions.

Finally, it is argued that surrogacy is harmful to women as a group. This objection is based on feminist concerns that the new reproductive technologies will increase the domination of men over women.[71] One envisioned feature of this increased domination is a continuing disintegration of the role of mother as we know it. More and more, women will be denied the role of *the* mother of their children, and will be placed in partial roles such as genetic, gestational, and social mother. An increase in these partial roles will mean a lessening of the individual woman's contribution to procreation. Thus, motherhood and apple pie will no longer mean what they do today (although apple pie probably will continue to be revered). The concern is that this trend will mean a loss of power and prestige for women. It seems unlikely, however, that surrogacy would have these negative consequences, if only because relatively few couples will have any of the three reasons stated above for entering surrogacy agreements. Few couples are infertile and have no other avenue for creating a child who is genetically related to at least one of them. Even fewer would seek surrogacy because of pregnancy-related health risks or for mere convenience. Thus, it is reasonable to believe that technology will separate the reproductive roles of women in only a small percentage of cases.

The above considerations support the fourth view, according to which commercial and noncommercial surrogacy should be permitted but regulated. A number of questions can be raised concerning the form that such regulation should take. What types of clauses should be permitted in surrogacy contracts? Should these contracts be legally enforceable? How should custody disputes be resolved if the surrogate changes her mind about relinquishing the child? The above discussion suggests some main points that can be made, as a step toward answering these questions.

First, regulations should include a requirement for screening and counseling of potential surrogate mothers. The aim would be to promote the informed consent of surrogates and to identify, if possible, those who seem to be at especially high risk of later deciding to keep the child. Second, payments that are contingent on live birth should not be allowed, both to protect the surrogate and to prevent surrogacy from being a form of baby selling. Third, clauses that require the surrogate to undergo amniocentesis and abortion should not be allowed. These matters can, of course, be discussed prior to entering the surrogacy contract. Selection of a surrogate by the commissioning couple can be based in part on her professed views concerning these matters. However, she should not be required to undergo these procedures. Fourth, at least some provisions of surrogacy contracts should be legally enforceable. For example, if the commissioning couple fails to pay the fee, then the surrogate mother should be able to seek a legal remedy, and the court should award her the contract price. Similarly, if the couple refuses to accept the child and the surrogate mother puts the child up for adoption, she should be able to seek compensation for costs incurred as a result of the adoption. Fifth, clauses requiring the surrogate to relinquish the child should not be legally enforceable. If she changes her mind about relinquishing, then the fact that she is the gestational mother — and in some cases the genetic mother, as well — suggests that she has at least a prima facie claim to a continuing involvement with the child and should be given an opportunity to present her case. If this is true, then her legal agreement to relinquish the child should not be the sole deciding factor. In other words, her prepregnancy agreement to relinquish the child should be considered legally *revokable.* If she does not wish to turn over the child, then a court should decide the issues of custody and visitation.

Various morally relevant factors should be considered by the court in making these decisions, perhaps the main ones being the well-being of the child and the relative abilities of the biological parents to raise the child. However, these factors might not always yield a definitive answer, in which case other morally relevant factors should be considered, including the prepregnancy intentions of the various parties and whether the surrogate is the genetic mother. In that event, the prepregnancy intentions as expressed in the surrogacy agreement should carry significant weight. Normally, this would result in a decision favoring the commissioning couple. The argument for giving priority to the commissioning couple is even stronger when the surrogate is not the genetic mother. This approach to decision making, based on morally relevant factors that can vary from case to case, follows the modified casuistic approach defended in Chapter 4. Sixth, if the surrogate relinquishes the child outright, then she should have no legal right to claim the child back. Once a stable family relationship is established, disrupting it might be too psychologically harmful to the child to justify a change in custody status.

We have considered arguments for and against three types of nontraditional family arrangements. In each case, the moral right to procreate has provided prima facie grounds for permitting such arrangements. Moreover, none of the objections to these arrangements are persuasive enough to justify the claim that the arrangements are morally wrong, much less that they should be legally prohibited. However, the arguments support the view that regulation of the process leading to nontraditional families sometimes is warranted, particularly in the case of surrogate motherhood.

6

Preembryos
Fertile Area for Bioethics

Several famous cases have raised issues concerning "frozen preembryos." The world took notice of frozen preembryos in 1983 when Mario and Elsa Rios died in an airplane crash, leaving behind two frozen preembryos in a Melbourne, Australia, in vitro fertilization clinic.[1] News stories focused on the Rios's substantial fortune and the question of whether the preembryos would be entitled to a share of the inheritance. Other issues were raised, as well: What should be done with the preembryos? Should they be donated to another infertile couple? Should they be discarded? Another case involved the divorce of Mary Sue and Junior Lewis Davis and their legal battle over seven frozen preembryos produced when they were IVF patients.[2] They had made no prior agreement concerning what to do with the preembryos in the event of divorce. Mary Sue initially wanted to transfer them to her uterus, but Junior stated that he no longer wanted her to have his children. The case revolved around a number of questions: What is the moral status of preembryos? Are they property? Who should decide their fate?

Disagreements over preembryos arise in other contexts, as well. An example is research involving preembryos, a topic addressed in a September 1994 report by a National Institutes of Health (NIH) advisory panel.[3] The report concluded that it is in the public interest for the NIH to fund research involving preembryos during the very early stages of development. However, some opponents expressed outrage. Jodie Brown, president of the American Life League, said her organization holds that a new life entitled to full human rights is created at conception, and that to use a fertilized egg for research "is murder."[4] A less strident but similar view is embodied in a Louisiana law passed in 1986, according to which a preembryo in vitro is legally a person.[5] The law states that it is illegal intentionally to destroy preembryos or to produce or maintain them in culture solely for research purposes.

Clearly, there are a number of issues that need to be addressed: What decisions are ethically justifiable concerning the creating, freezing, transferring, donating, researching, and discarding of preembryos, and who should make those decisions? In this chapter, the moral framework developed in Part 1 will be applied to these questions.

Developmental Process of the Preembryo

To address these issues, it is important to understand the biology involved. Although in Chapter 3 I briefly discussed some aspects of the development of preembryos, further description is needed to set the stage for discussion of the ethical issues. A lengthy and detailed description is not called for here, but it is necessary to identify some main features of preembryo development. In what follows, I draw upon helpful discussions by C. R. Austin and Clifford Grobstein.[6]

Fertilization, the combining of a sperm and oocyte, is a process, not an instantaneous event. It takes place over approximately a twenty-four-hour period following the sperm's penetration of the outer surface of the oocyte. Toward the end of this period, syngamy occurs, which is the coming together and aligning of the chromosomes of the oocyte and sperm. With syngamy, a new and unique genome forms. The fertilized egg, or zygote, is a single cell. The early cell divisions are referred to as "cleavage" because the cells become smaller with each division. The individual cells are called blastomeres. Until about the eight-cell stage, the cells are totipotent, meaning that each cell, if separated, is capable of developing into a whole individual. Twins can be formed if there is a splitting of the cell mass.[7] Freezing of preembryos typically is carried out at the one- to eight-cell stage.[8]

At about four to five days following fertilization, a fluid-filled central cavity forms within the cell mass, at which point the preembryo is called a blastocyst. Normally, the blastocyst is in the uterus at this time but unattached to the uterine lining. At this point, differentiation of cells is under way, and it is possible to distinguish a peripheral cell layer and an inner cell mass. The peripheral cells are attaining the ability to interact with maternal cells of the uterine lining and will develop into structures that are the forerunners of the placenta and amniotic membrane. The inner cell mass is the part that will develop into the embryo proper. At approximately six to nine days, the blasto-cyst becomes implanted in the uterus. By the tenth day it usually is completely embedded within the uterine lining. At this point, pregnancy is regarded as established. Without implantation, the preembryo will not develop to any significant degree beyond this point because maternal cells contribute in a cru-cial way, currently not well understood, to its ongoing development.[9] More-over, if a preembryo is cultured in vitro beyond the stage at which interaction with the uterine lining usually takes place and then is transferred to a uterus, it will not implant.

During approximately ten to fourteen days following fertilization, the inner cell mass is forming two distinct cell layers. At first these layers are shaped roughly as a circular disc, but they progressively become ovoid. At about the fourteenth day, a darker-colored linear streak appears along the long axis of the ovoid, beginning at one end. This end will be the hind-end of the em-bryonic axis and the opposite will be the fore-end, where development of the head eventually will occur. This dark line is called the primitive streak. Some-times one streak appears, indicating that there will be a singleton pregnancy. Less often, two streaks appear, indicating twins. Twinning also can occur when for some reason the inner cell mass divides into distinct parts, but the appearance of the primitive streak is considered to be the latest point at which twinning can take place and marks the beginning of the embryo proper. The embryonic period is defined as extending from the beginning of the third week until the end of the eighth week following fertilization. At the beginning of the ninth week, the term *fetus* is used.

The above discussion reveals several reasons why the distinction between preembryos and embryos is important. First, it is the embryonic disc contain-ing a primitive streak — not the peripheral cell layer — that has the potential to become a self-conscious individual. Because the preembryo as a whole is not identical to the embryonic disc, it lacks the potential to *become* self-conscious and possesses only the potential to *cause* self-consciousness.[10] Thus, there is a morally relevant difference between preembryos and embryos, although I ar-gued in Chapter 3 that this difference is not large. Second, the fact that de-velopment beyond the implantation stage cannot currently be accomplished in vitro means that it is not possible to create *embryos* extracorporally at present. Thus, *all* of the activities at issue, including freezing, donating, discarding, research, and so on, currently are carried out on preembryos, not embryos.

Moral Status of Preembryos

In Chapter 3 I presented a view concerning the moral status of pre-embryos, embryos, and fetuses. According to that view, some degree of conferred moral standing is justifiable for certain individuals that are not descriptive persons, based on consequentialist considerations. I argued that the degree of conferred moral standing increases during pregnancy, as the number of morally relevant similarities to the paradigm of descriptive persons increases. The argument for conferred moral standing for preembryos is relatively weak because they have only one morally relevant similarity, the potential to cause self-consciousness. Preembryos should be treated with some degree of respect because failure to do so could have adverse consequences for persons in the descriptive sense. However, the amount of respect called for is far less than that owed to descriptive persons.

A more thorough defense of my view requires consideration of alternative viewpoints. As pointed out in a report by the American Society for Reproductive Medicine, three main views concerning the moral status of preembryos have been put forward.[11] One view is that preembryos have the status of normative personhood. This view usually is based on a religious belief that personhood begins at conception. The Roman Catholic church, for example, has stated such a view in its official writings.[12] There seem to be two versions of the argument that personhood begins at conception. One version holds that because prenatal development is gradual and continuous, there is no special point during gestation at which it can reasonably be said that personhood begins. Therefore, the only point that could plausibly mark the beginning of personhood is conception because it is the only discontinuity — a new individual comes into being with the union of sperm and ovum.[13] The second version states that there is uncertainty concerning when personhood begins. To avoid the risk of destroying persons, it is argued, we should regard personhood as beginning at conception, the earliest point at which it plausibly could occur.[14]

In explaining what is wrong with these arguments, several points deserve mention. First, both versions assume that there is a point during prenatal development at which personhood begins. They overlook the alternative view that moral standing increases as development proceeds during gestation. Thus, they are based on a fundamental assumption that is not defended. By contrast, the view that moral standing increases during gestation is supported by sound arguments, as outlined in Chapter 3. Second, the view that personhood begins at conception leads to implausible conclusions in specific cases. Consider the example discussed in Chapter 3: a fire breaks out in a laboratory, and you must choose between rescuing a preembryo or a ten-year-old child.

According to the view in question, both are persons in the normative sense and it is morally justifiable to rescue either one. However, clearly it would be morally wrong to select the preembryo over the child. The view that moral standing increases during gestation yields the correct conclusion in this case and is consistent with other widely held moral intuitions, including the following: use of intrauterine devices for birth control seems morally acceptable, even though they cause the nonimplantation and death of preembryos; and abortion early in gestation is less problematic ethically than late abortion.

A second main view is that preembryos have the same status as any other human tissue. The problem with this view is that it overlooks the argument for some degree of conferred moral status based on the preembryo's potential to cause self-consciousness. Others have replied to this second view by stating that the preembryo has *symbolic value* — that it is a symbol of human life. I suggest that the best way to understand such replies is to regard them as consequentialist arguments, to the effect that adverse consequences will occur if the symbol is not respected. Thus, my account of conferred moral standing is consistent with, and is a way of understanding, the view that preembryos have symbolic value.

The third view takes an intermediate position. It holds that preembryos are not persons but deserve special respect. The view I defended in Chapter 3 is a version of this approach. However, this view raises several questions: What does it *mean* to give respect to a preembryo? To what extent should preembryos be given respect? Our moral framework suggests an approach to answering these questions. It maintains that the preembryo's moral status is based on consequentialist considerations. In deciding whether particular actions should be carried out in order to show respect for preembryos, we therefore should consider the consequences of performing and not performing those actions. Some possible ways of showing respect toward preembryos will be considered in this chapter.

Who Should Decide?

There is a strong ethical argument for the view that the progenitors, the persons whose oocyte and sperm formed the preembryo, should have decision-making authority concerning it. They should decide because the decision will significantly affect their interests in ways the interests of others will not be affected. I am referring, of course, to their reproductive interests, the most basic of which are their interests in procreating and not procreating. In Chapter 1, I discussed some of the main reasons why procreating can be meaningful to persons. In the present context, procreation would involve "assisted reproduction" rather than coitus. Despite this fact, a number of the reasons identified in Chapter 1 for valuing procreation would be applicable. Some might regard such procreation as important in part because it involves participation in the creation of a person. For others, it might be valued as an affirmation of mutual love. Some will desire it as a link to future persons, and it can result in important experiences of pregnancy, childbirth, and child rearing. These are reasons for allowing the progenitors to decide whether their preembryos will be used in an attempt to procreate. Also, we have considered the suffering that infertility can cause. Giving infertile couples decisional authority over their preembryos can help reduce this suffering when their decisions result in the birth of a child. Moreover, freedom to procreate and freedom not to procreate are important to self-identity, self-fulfillment, and self-determination. The rights to procreate and not to procreate, for which I argued earlier, imply a prima facie right of progenitors to decisional authority over their preembryos. Thus, there is a presumption that the progenitors should make the decisions, unless their right to do so is overridden by other ethical concerns.

These considerations support the view that the progenitors have a prima facie right to use preembryos for their own reproductive purposes, to authorize the freezing of them, to donate them to other infertile couples, to donate them for research, or to destroy them, if that is their wish. The prima facie right to destroy or discard their preembryos is not overridden by the preembryos' moral status because, as I argued, that status is relatively low. In the event of the death of one of the progenitors, the right to make the decisions would continue to be held by the surviving progenitor.

A recent legal case, *York v. Jones,* resulted in a ruling that is consistent with the above ethical analysis.[15] That case involved Risa Adler-York and Steven York, who became infertility patients in 1986 at the Howard and Georgeanna Jones Institute for Reproductive Medicine in Norfolk, Virginia. Subsequently, the Yorks moved to Los Angeles but continued being patients at the Jones Institute. On four occasions they returned to Norfolk for IVF procedures. All four IVF attempts were unsuccessful, but the fourth produced an extra preembryo that was frozen for later use. In 1988 they enrolled as infertility patients at the Hospital of the Good Samaritan in Los Angeles. They asked the Jones Institute to release the frozen preembryo for shipment to Los Angeles, where it would be thawed and placed in Risa's uterus by their new infertility doctor. However, the Norfolk program refused to turn over the preembryo, and the couple then sued in federal district court in Norfolk to obtain custody of it. The court ruled in favor of the Yorks, finding it reasonable for them to claim a legal right to make the decisions concerning the preembryo and to claim a right to immediate possession.

To say that the progenitors should be the ones to decide entails, of course, that their choices should be made voluntarily. An important point made by feminist writers is that women undergoing IVF can be subjected to pressures that impede voluntariness.[16] Sources of social pressure to reproduce can include male partners, family, friends, and the health professionals specializing in infertility treatment. It is important for the health professionals to be sensitive to these pressures and to help promote the voluntariness of choices by women as well as men who are infertility patients.

Should Preembryos Be Regarded as Property?

Given that the progenitors should make the decisions, should we say that preembryos are their property? To answer this question, it is important to distinguish two senses of the term *property*. It is commonly used to refer to a "thing" or "object" that is owned. In law, however, property is regarded as the collection of *legal rights* that exist concerning the thing. These are rights, of one or more individuals, to control and make decisions about the object in question. They include the right to possess the thing, to exclude others from possessing and interfering with it, to dispose of it by gift or sale, to use it, to enjoy the fruits and profits derived from it, and to destroy it.[17] Thus, in legal language, to say that progenitors have a property interest in their preembryos is just to say that they have the decisional authority concerning possession, use, destruction, and so on. This property language has been used in court cases involving preembryos; in *York v. Jones,* for example, the judge referred to the Yorks' right to decide as a property interest.[18]

In discussing the ethics of decision making about preembryos, however, it is not necessary to use the language of property. All the ethically relevant concerns can be expressed without referring to the preembryo as property and without using the expression "property interest." The interests that progenitors have in making decisions can be expressed in terms of their interests in reproductive freedom. Consider, for example, the York case. We can say that the Yorks should make the decisions concerning use, storage, transfer, and so on, because of the implications such decisions have for their freedom to procreate and freedom not to procreate.

It might be objected that it sometimes is necessary to use the term "property," particularly if the decision about preembryos does not directly involve reproduction. To consider another example, suppose that the Yorks had wanted to send the preembryo to another research center where it would be used for research and then discarded, and the Jones Institute refused this request. It might be claimed that the only way the Yorks could assert their rights in this context would be to assert a property interest, because the shipping of the preembryo would not affect whether they reproduced. However, it can be argued that the progenitors' reproductive freedom justifies their controlling this type of decision as well. If others gain de facto control, the preembryos might be used, whether intentionally or unintentionally, in ways that have reproductive consequences for the progenitors. Reproduction using the preembryos might be carried out or foreclosed, against the progenitors' wishes. To protect against preembryos being used against their wishes in ways that have reproductive consequences for them, the progenitors should have thorough dispositional control. Thus, even in the hypothetical scenario being considered, we can discuss the ethical aspects of decision making without using the term "property."

Furthermore, there are reasons supporting the view that we should avoid referring to preembryos as property and avoid terms like "property interest" which carry the connotation that preembryos are property. As two commentators have put it: "There is a qualitative difference between the preembryo and other 'things' recognized as property. . . . One may wonder whether the property . . . approach can be limited so the preembryo does not become an ordinary thing or object. Ideas are powerful; and, once the preembryo is defined as some kind of property, it will be difficult to avoid the implications of property law."[19] Regarding preembryos as property seems inconsistent with the idea that at least some degree of respect should be given. Respect implies that there are limits to what we may do with them. However, if they are property, then it seems that owners can do whatever they wish to them. The question was raised above concerning what might be involved in treating preembryos with "respect." One way to show respect — to acknowledge they they have at least *some* moral status — is to avoid labeling them as "property" and, whenever possible, to avoid the language of property rights and property interests in regard to them.

However, it must be admitted that the language of property is entrenched in the law. As a practical matter, in courtroom argumentation concerning preembryos, sometimes it might not be feasible to avoid referring to property rights and interests. We might say, then, that one way to show respect for preembryos is to refrain from using the language of property in regard to them unless it is reasonably unavoidable.

This discussion has implications for the question of whether it is ethical to buy and sell preembryos. To exchange money or anything of value for preembryos is to treat them as property that may be bought and sold. I suggest that another appropriate way to acknowledge that preembryos have at least some moral standing is to avoid buying and selling them, and even legally to forbid such buying and selling. This is not meant to imply, however, that it is wrong to compensate sperm, oocyte, or preembryo donors for the time, inconvenience, discomforts, or risks involved in donation.

Freezing Preembryos

Use of superovulatory drugs often results in the formation of multiple preembryos, sometimes as many as ten or more. However, it is preferable to transfer a smaller number — usually at most four or five — during any one cycle, in order to reduce the risk of multiple gestation. Most IVF programs freeze the extra preembryos to save them for use in future cycles, in the event pregnancy is not achieved in the first cycle. Thus, freezing provides an opportunity to increase the pregnancy rate per retrieval. The ethical justification of freezing is that it facilitates the efforts of the infertile couple to have children by in vitro fertilization. It does this by avoiding the need to have an oocyte retrieval for every transfer cycle, thereby eliminating the associated costs, inconvenience, discomfort, and risks to the woman.[20]

However, objections have been raised against freezing preembryos. First, there is concern that freezing might kill some preembryos. This objection is stated in *Donum Vitae*: "*The freezing of embryos*, even when carried out in order to preserve the life of an embryo — cryopreservation — *constitutes an offense against the respect due to human beings* by exposing them to grave risks of death or harm to their physical integrity."[21] Available evidence indicates that 30 to 48 percent of preembryos do not survive freezing and thawing.[22] However, we do not know the extent to which freezing contributes to this loss. Even when there is no freezing, a substantial proportion of preembryos do not survive to the blastocyst stage.[23] Although freezing might contribute to preembryo loss, the alternative usually would be to discard the extra preembryos. Immediate donation to another infertile couple typically would not be feasible because synchronization of menstrual cycles would be required. Thus, the concern that preembryos should not be killed, assuming it were valid, would be served better by freezing because that gives them a chance for survival.

A second objection to freezing is based on a more general objection to any manipulations that contribute to the separation of reproduction and sexual intercourse. This objection also is put forward in *Donum Vitae* and is based on the religious belief that it is wrong to separate these two activities.[24] Freezing contributes to this separation because it facilitates noncoital reproduction. In reply, it should be pointed out that the objection is based on a religious claim that it is God's judgment that a certain type of action is wrong. No additional ethical argument is given that is independent of this religious claim.[25] The claim itself rests ultimately on religious faith, as opposed to reasoned arguments. However, professional ethics and public policy in a pluralistic society should be grounded on reasoned arguments, rather than religious beliefs alone, for at least two reasons. The first is the simple fact that many persons do not subscribe to the religious beliefs in question. The second and perhaps more fundamental reason is that professional ethics and public policy should be rationally justifiable, but religious beliefs accepted as a matter of faith do not seem to reach this level of justification.

Third, it might be objected that freezing could cause birth defects. Here the ethical concern is focused not on the preembryos themselves but on the children who might come into being. In reply, preembryo freezing has been used extensively in farm animals and laboratory mice with no evidence of an increased rate of birth defects.[26] Although this is reassuring, it is not clear whether the results of animal studies carry over to the human species. In humans, however, the number of live births following freezing and thawing of preembryos has increased with the growing use of cryopreservation. At present, no data has been published to show that there is a statistically significant increase in the rate of birth defects as a result of freezing.

Donation of Preembryos

There are several types of situations in which an infertile couple might want to receive donated preembryos. One is the relatively infrequent situation in which there are medical indications both for donor oocytes and for donor sperm. Second, if there is an indication for donor oocytes but none are available, a couple might consider receiving donor preembryos. Third, in cases of male infertility where the man objects to donor insemination, the couple might consider receiving preembryos.

The ethical argument for preembryo donation is that it enables some infertile couples to have a child. Several of the reasons for valuing procreation are relevant in this context: because the infertile woman would be the gestational mother, assuming one or more donated preembryos implanted, she would have experiences associated with pregnancy and childbirth; she would participate in the creation of a person; and she and her partner would be given the opportunity for experiences associated with child rearing.

However, objections to preembryo donation have been raised by the Catholic church. One objection is based on the religious belief that God considers use of third-party gametes in reproduction to be wrong.[27] I responded to this type of religious objection above, in discussing preembryo freezing. The problems with the objection are the same as discussed before: many persons do not hold the religious beliefs in question; and public policy and professional ethics should be rationally justifiable.

Additional objections are found in *Donum Vitae*'s discussion of "hetero-logous artificial fertilization," which refers to techniques using gametes coming from at least one donor other than the two spouses joined in marriage: "Heterologous artificial fertilization violates the rights of the child; it deprives him of his filial relationship with his parental origins and can hinder the maturing of his personal identity."[28] Two arguments can be identified in this passage. First, heterologous artificial fertilization, which includes preembryo donation, violates the right of children to have a filial relationship with their genetic parents. Second, it harms the children because depriving them of this filial relationship hinders the maturing of their personal identity.

In response to the first argument, it is not obvious that there is such a right. Even if we grant that it is desirable, other things being equal, that children be raised from birth by their genetic parents, it does not necessarily follow that alternative rearing arrangements violate any right of the child. This raises the question of how one would establish that there is such a right. My analysis of rights in Chapter 1 suggests that we should ask the following question: Does bringing children into being in circumstances involving rearing arrangements that deprive them of filial relationships with their genetic parents amount to treating them as mere means and not as ends in themselves? If so, then we have grounds for saying that a right is violated. However, it is not clear that such arrangements fail to treat children as ends in themselves. The children in question would not exist except for preembryo donation, given that the donating couple does not wish to transfer the preembryo to the donor woman's uterus. The fact that such children are given life makes it possible for them to become ends in themselves. If the children are loved, nurtured, and treated with due respect, it would seem odd to say that they are not being treated as ends in themselves. In reply to the second argument, the same mistake is made concerning the concept of harm that I discussed in Chapter 5. If it were not for heterologous artificial fertilization, the children in question would not exist. The objection therefore amounts to saying that the children conceived in this manner are worse off than they would have been if they had not been conceived. However, being raised by persons other than genetic parents does not constitute having a life in which pain and suffering outweigh any positive experiences that might occur. Thus, the objection should be rejected.

A further objection is found in *Donum Vitae*. In a discussion of the rupture between genetic, gestational, and social parenthood, the following statement is made: "Such damage to the personal relationships within the family has repercussions on civil society: What threatens the unity and stability of the family is a source of dissension, disorder, and injustice in the whole of social life."[29] I agree that threats to the unity and stability of the family as an institution would be matters of grave concern. However, does collaborative reproduction really pose such a threat? The objection envisions a future in which the traditional family, involving two heterosexual nondivorcing parents with children, will have disintegrated. There are several reasons for doubting that collaborative reproduction would contribute significantly to such an outcome. First, only a small percentage of couples are infertile and would need to resort to collaborative reproduction to have children. For the most part, people will continue to form families without using third-party gametes or preembryos. Second, in an important sense, third-party collaboration is promotive of families, in that it enables families to come into being. Admittedly, they do not have the traditional form referred to above, but they are just as capable of forming the basis of family life and sustaining important values associated with family. At present, claims that collaborative reproduction will lead to dissolution of the family seem too speculative to justify the view that such collaboration ethically is wrong or that it should be prohibited.

Research Using Preembryos

Is research using preembryos ethically permissible? A widely held view is that most research using preembryos is unethical and should be prohibited. Ireland and Germany, for example, have made it illegal to carry out all preembryo research except that which promotes the "interests" of the preembryos upon which the research is performed.[30] A problem with such laws, of course, is that preembryos lack interests because they are not sentient. Similar restrictions on "nontherapeutic" research are found in South Australia; and a Louisiana statute states, "No in vitro fertilized human ovum will be . . . cultured solely for research purposes."[31]

However, many areas of medicine can be identified in which "nontherapeutic" preembryo research promises to give us important knowledge. To appreciate the extent of this potential knowledge, let us consider some examples. One area is male infertility in which fertilization cannot be achieved in vitro because the sperm count is too low or the sperm have fertilization defects. A technique being developed to deal with this problem is microinjection, in which a single sperm is injected under the zona pellucida (the outer membrane of the oocyte) or directly into the cytoplasm of the oocyte. One concern is whether this technique might produce chromosomal abnormalities. Thus, it would be desirable to observe the effects of the technique on the development of the fertilized ovum before it is offered as a treatment. However, this would involve creating, observing, and then discarding preembryos.[32]

In addition, there is a need for research to improve the success rate of IVF. In terms of live births, the current success rate is 15 to 25 percent per cycle of oocyte collection. To put it differently, about three out of each hundred oocytes collected will result in a live birth.[33] Improved techniques can be discovered only if new approaches are compared to those used previously. Areas of study include different drugs for superovulation and different culture media, among others. Trying out new approaches, of course, amounts to research using preembryos.

Research into improved cryopreservation is also desirable. Approximately 30 to 48 percent of preembryos that are frozen and thawed do not survive.[34] Improvements would include better freezing methods and identification of nonviable preembryos prior to freezing. Discovery of improved methods unavoidably involves trying them with preembryos. Freezing of oocytes also is an area being investigated. One question is whether freezing oocytes damages their chromosomes. Study of chromosomal injuries might be facilitated by fertilizing thawed oocytes in vitro, allowing them to develop, and testing the preembryos genetically.[35]

Another area is research into early pregnancy loss. Many pregnancies fail at very early stages of gestation, and the exact causes are unknown. Possibly in some cases the cause is failure of cells to differentiate properly into specialized cells. Research into the process of cell differentiation, which occurs in the preembryo, might some day help prevent some cases of early pregnancy loss.[36]

Discovery of improved methods of contraception would be a welcomed advance. One possible approach is contraceptive vaccines.[37] Such vaccines would target a specific antigen necessary for fertilization or early development. For example, sperm are covered with antigens that are believed to play a role in functions such as sperm movement and attachment to oocytes. The purpose of a vaccine would be to produce antibodies that block the biological function of a given antigen. Thus, if anti-sperm antibodies could be produced, they would attach to spermatozoa and neutralize their potential for fertilization either by reducing their motility or disrupting their capacity to fertilize the ovum. Clinical trials of such vaccines might involve certain risks: if the vaccine fails, an unwanted pregnancy could occur; possibly there would be an abnormality in the child thus produced, caused by the vaccine. Thus, prior to clinical trials, it would be desirable to test the antibodies in vitro and determine, if they fail, the normalcy of the preembryos produced. Another approach to im-

proved contraception would be to learn more about the process of implantation, possibly leading to the discovery of drugs or antibodies that block that
phase of development.

Preimplantation detection of genetic abnormalities is an area of ongoing
research. A blastomere can be removed from an early preembryo and tested
for genetic defects. Detection of preembryos carrying the cystic fibrosis gene
has already been reported.[38] Tests to detect other genetic defects in preembryos undoubtedly will be possible in the future. Such testing is desirable
because it helps couples avoid having children with serious genetic diseases.

Cancer research is another worthy area of study involving preembryos.
There is evidence that certain genes involved in causing cancer, called proto-
oncogenes, play a role in cell differentiation. Some of these genes might be
involved in the normal process of preembryo and embryo development. Study
of their normal function in the preembryo might promote our understanding
of the role they play in the development of cancer.[39]

Finally, new types of transplantation could arise from study of stem cells.
These are the cells that give rise to the differentiated, or specialized, cells
required for the development of organs and tissues. Stem cells could be obtained from preembryos or embryos in the early post-implantation stage of
development. Cells that produce blood, called hematopoietic stem cells, might
prove useful in treating serious blood diseases such as leukemia and many
anemias. Preembryo and embryo cells do not have the immunologic properties
that lead to rejection in transplantation. Thus, therapy consisting of intra-
venous injection of embryonic hematopoietic stem cells could be carried out
without the need for immunosuppressive drugs or tissue matching.[40] Such an
approach might be more effective and produce a better quality of life for
transplant recipients than current therapies.

These potential medical benefits provide reasons for allowing preembryo
research to go forward. Moreover, laws prohibiting "nontherapeutic" research reflect a mistaken view of the ethics of preembryo research. Such laws
typically are based on the view that preembryos deserve the same protections
as persons. The ethical framework developed in this book helps to show why
that view is wrong. The main point is that preembryos have a relatively low
degree of moral standing. They are not persons in the normative or descriptive
senses, so the moral rules concerning persons as research subjects are not
directly applicable. Of course, informed consent should be obtained from
persons who donate preembryos for research, and guidelines are needed because of possible consequences of preembryo research for society. Within such
constraints, research conducted with sound scientific design and that promises
to yield valuable information can be justified on the grounds that the benefits

to be gained outweigh any reasonable concerns based on the preembryo's moral status.

Objections to research using preembryos come mainly from two sources — religious groups such as the Catholic church and certain feminists. I have responded to the religious arguments, so let me focus now on feminist objections. It should be pointed out that not all feminists object to preembryo research, although a significant number of them do. An example is Robyn Rowland, who identifies several women-centered concerns arising from such research.[41] First, producing preembryos can involve significant risks to women, such as risks associated with superovulation drugs. Second, there is pressure to use new techniques and to participate in research, and this compromises the voluntariness of consent by women.[42]

Other feminist objections, raised by Rowland and others,[43] are based on broader concerns about the new reproductive technologies as a whole. They arise from the view that reproductive technologies will increase the domination of men over women. As women are denied the role of *the* mother of their children, it is claimed, there will be a devaluation of motherhood, an associated loss of power for women, and increased commodification of the woman's contribution to procreation. This view is expressed vividly by Gena Corea, who draws a comparison to prostitution: "While sexual prostitutes sell vagina, rectum and mouth, reproductive-prostitutes will sell other body parts: wombs; ovaries; eggs."[44]

This objection paints a powerful image, and it alerts us to a possible outcome that must be avoided. Concern about the impact of our policies on women as a group is important, and it is often overlooked in discussions of bioethics. Nevertheless, the specific objection in question significantly overstates the likely negative consequences of reproductive technologies, as I pointed out in Chapter 5 in discussing surrogate motherhood. Only a small percentage of couples are infertile. Although reproductive technologies might be used by couples who are not infertile, perhaps for convenience or other reasons, the number who would do so is likely to be small because of the high costs involved. It is reasonable to believe that technology will separate the reproductive roles of women in only a small percentage of cases.

However, ethical guidelines for preembryo research should reflect a concern about its potential impact on women and should include the following points: women should participate in any process of setting forth national policies concerning preembryo research; and the likely impact of any proposed national policies upon women as a group should be an important consideration in their assessment. It is worth noting that the recent report of the NIH Human Embryo Research Panel does not include these points as explicit guidelines.[45]

Ethical guidelines also should include the requirement that the informed consent of those whose gametes form the preembryos should be obtained prior to the research being carried out. The concern raised by Rowland is important, and women should be adequately informed of any risks they are asked to undertake. Furthermore, clinicians must be sensitive to the pressures on infertile couples to participate in research.

Additional guidelines should address at least three issues: Is it ethical for preembryos used in research to be replaced in a woman's uterus? Is it permissible to create preembryos solely for research purposes? To what developmental stage may preembryos (or embryos) be maintained in the laboratory? Let us turn to these questions.

REPLACEMENT OF PREEMBRYOS

Replacing preembryos used in research to a woman's uterus raises the concern that research manipulations might injure the child who is born. Some have claimed that, to avoid such injury, preembryos used in research should never be replaced in a uterus.[46] However, this would mean that some important types of research could not be carried out. For example, research on preimplantation genetic testing would be ruled out because it involves replacement of preembryos with normal test results to the woman's uterus. Similarly, research that aims to improve IVF success rates, such as comparisons of different culture media, would be eliminated. It seems better to permit such research provided the following two conditions are met: replacement to a woman's uterus is a necessary component of the research; and available evidence makes it reasonable to believe that the research will not cause an injury.[47]

CREATING PREEMBRYOS SOLELY FOR RESEARCH

Some believe that it is wrong to create preembryos solely for research purposes. This view has resulted in laws against such creation in some European countries, including Ireland, Germany, and Spain, in the state of Victoria in Australia, and in Louisiana.[48] The usual argument for this view is that preembryos have substantial moral standing and that creating them solely for research treats them as mere means. However, this argument is mistaken because it assumes that the preembryo is an end in itself. A more defensible view is that only a relatively small degree of moral status should be conferred upon the preembryo, as I have argued.

Even though preembryos have only a small degree of moral status, it might be asked whether "respect" for preembryos requires that they not be created solely for research purposes. As stated above, the question of what should be done to show respect for preembryos should be resolved on the basis of consequentialist considerations. This would include consideration of the advancement of scientific knowledge. Prohibiting the creation of preembryos solely for research purposes prevents some types of important research. For example, the chromosomal studies of frozen oocytes mentioned above would be barred. This would inhibit the development of oocyte freezing, a technique that might some day largely replace preembryo freezing in IVF programs.[49] Similarly, important aspects of the study of microinjection would be precluded. For example, it would not be possible to observe the development of microinjected ova into preembryos or to test the preembryos for chromosomal normality.[50] It seems reasonable to believe that the benefits of research outweigh any adverse consequences associated with creating preembryos solely for research. Respect for preembryos does not require that we refrain from creating them for such purposes.

TIME LIMIT FOR CULTURE

To what developmental stage may preembryos (or embryos) be maintained extracorporally? Many committee reports have advocated a limit at fourteen days following fertilization,[51] and some countries such as Great Britain[52] and Spain[53] have passed laws establishing a limit at fourteen days. The argument that has been advanced for the fourteen-day limit is that an individual does not exist prior to the formation of the primitive streak, which appears at about fourteen days. This argument was a response to the view that ensoulment begins at conception and that preembryos therefore deserve protection. The basis of the argument is the fact that twinning can occur up to the formation of the primitive streak. Twinning undermines the ensoulment-at-conception theory because one must explain what happens to the soul when twinning occurs. It either divides into two or a second soul appears, but both explanations are inconsistent with the doctrine that souls are indivisible and created at conception. Thus, it is argued, the earliest an individual can exist is at fourteen days because ensoulment cannot plausibly occur before then. By drawing the line at fourteen days, it is claimed, we are assured of not doing research on ensouled entities.

This response to the ensoulment-at-conception theory supports the view that there should be no limit prior to fourteen days, but we should also consider whether a limit that extends beyond fourteen days would be reasonable. In deciding where the limit should be, we need to consider why it is desirable to establish a limit. I suggest that a limit at *some* point is needed because we can envision a possible future in which embryos can be maintained extracorporally longer and longer. We can envision, perhaps with horror, embryos and fetuses being grown in the laboratory so they can be studied and then discarded. At *some* stage of development, being maintained in this way is inconsistent with the moral status of the entity being studied. Establishing a line helps to prevent this sort of ethically unjustifiable research.

Let us consider the following scenario: We learn that a group of scientists have carried out research that involved keeping embryos alive in vitro up to twenty-one days following fertilization, after which they discarded them. We learn also that the research was scientifically important and performed in a jurisdiction that does not legally forbid such research, so no laws were broken. Should we consider such research unethical simply because it extended past fourteen days? The answer, I believe, is no. A twenty-one-day embryo should have only a relatively small degree of conferred moral standing. It lacks viability, sentience, and any physical resemblance to paradigmatic persons. The research in question would not be inconsistent with its moral status. But if there is nothing sacrosanct about fourteen days, where should the line be drawn?

Different authors have suggested different places to draw the line. Helga Kuhse and Peter Singer have expressed the view that destructive experimentation would be ethical any time before the acquiring of sentience.[54] Prior to sentience, they argue, the embryo or fetus has no interests and therefore would not be harmed by research followed by destruction. The problem with their view is that it overlooks the grounds for conferred moral standing for the fetus prior to sentience. It has been suggested that sentience could not occur prior to about twenty to twenty-four weeks of gestation.[55] Fetuses at a stage just prior to this have several morally relevant similarities to paradigmatic persons, including physical resemblance and the potential to become self-conscious. Destructive research with such advanced fetuses would not appear to be consistent with their conferred moral status.[56] Another view, put forward by Hans-Martin Sass, is that destructive research may be carried out prior to the beginning of active brain functioning such as "organ control, central coordination, and interactive connection" between brain parts.[57] He suggests that until we know more about when exactly such brain function begins, the fiftieth day after menstruation would be a "morally very comfortable and safe" line to prevent research on embryos with brain function as defined.[58] The problem with this view is that the onset of "brain function," as defined by Sass, does not have any special moral significance. He thinks it is significant because he uses a mistaken analogy with brain death. He reasons that if life ends when brain death occurs, then moral recognition and legal protection of human life should begin when brain function begins. This reasoning fails to appreciate the distinction between necessary and sufficient conditions. From the concept of brain death it only follows that brain activity is a *necessary* condition for life — when brain activity ceases irreversibly, life ceases. It does not follow that brain activity is a sufficient condition for morally recognized and legally protected life. Sass's view should be rejected.

I suggest that a more plausible line is somewhere in the mid-embryonic period, before the embryo begins to acquire a more human-like appearance. I believe that it clearly would be unacceptable to maintain the entity until the beginning of the fetal period, at which point there is a distinct human-like appearance. This appearance constitutes an important similarity with paradigmatic persons that the early embryo lacks. Although some have maintained that physical appearance is not morally relevant, I have argued that it is, and I believe it can provide a basis for drawing a line somewhere in the mid-embryonic period — that is, somewhere from the end of the fourth to the end of the sixth week after fertilization.

There are several reasons why the fourteen-day limit has become so widely accepted. First, the formation of the primitive streak has *some* moral significance, because it marks the coming into being of an individual having the potential to *become* self-conscious. Second, it fulfills the need for there to be *some* limit on how long preembryos and embryos may be maintained in the laboratory. Third, it does not interfere with *any* current research because it is not now possible to maintain preembryos in vitro to fourteen days.[59] However, the fourteen-day limit does not accurately reflect our considered opinions concerning the stage of development at which maintaining the entity becomes unjustifiable. Also, the moral difference between the preembryo and early embryo is not great enough to establish fourteen days as a line that must never be crossed. In addition, some types of valuable research might some day be possible that would require crossing the fourteen-day line. An example would be research involving embryonic stem cells, referred to above. In conclusion, the fourteen-day rule might be reasonable at present because of the reasons identified above. However, the fact that this rule has become so widely accepted suggests that it might become "carved in stone," and I believe this would be a mistake.

Blastomere Separation

Blastomere separation is a technique that might help increase the success rate of IVF. It involves removing the zona pellucida from an early preembryo, separating the preembryo into its constituent cells, and covering the cells with an artificial zona pellucida. The result is the creation of several duplicates of the original preembryo. Blastomere separation has been used in cattle breeding, but only recently has there been interest in applying it to human pre-embryos. A step toward blastomere separation using human preembryos was accomplished when Jerry L. Hall and colleagues carried out the technique using polyploid human preembryos.[60] These are preembryos formed when an oocyte is fertilized by more than one sperm. They have more than the normal number of chromosomes and are not viable, but are capable of dividing and staying alive for a short period. Hall used polyploid preembryos because they are not clinically usable.

In applying blastomere separation to IVF, the idea is to create additional preembryos so more will be available for transfer. This might be particularly useful when only a few preembryos are produced following oocyte retrieval. If effective, it might increase the number of live births per retrieval cycle. Whether the technique would work is unknown. Some have expressed the view that it might not be as helpful as initially thought. If failure to implant is sometimes caused by genetic defects, then duplicating genetically defective preembryos will not improve IVF success rates.[61] Nevertheless, duplicating genetically normal preembryos might increase success rates.

Hall and his coworkers mistakenly referred to their experiment as cloning.[62] The term *cloning* refers to a different process that involves removing the nucleus from a cell of an adult and placing it in an oocyte whose own nucleus has been removed. When successful, the result is an individual who is genetically identical to the original adult.[63] Robert J. Stillman, one of Hall's coauthors, stated that they used "cloning" in a broader sense according to which a clone is an identical replication, a duplicate copy.[64] However, what they did was not cloning even in this broad sense because polyploid cells do not produce genetically identical daughter cells when they divide.[65] Their experiment was not cloning and should not be called cloning.[66]

Cloning, in the sense involving nucleus transfer, raises a number of ethical issues because it entails the possibility of engineering humans and making many copies of them. These issues include whether the lack of uniqueness of the individuals produced would be psychologically harmful to them and whether it is likely that engineering that is harmful to society would occur. In blastomere separation, by contrast, only a few duplicates can be produced.[67] Thus, these ethical issues raised by cloning do not easily transfer to blastomere separation because it does not carry the same potential for engineering. The reason blastomere separation should not be called cloning is that doing so creates the mistaken impression that it can be used to engineer humans in a way similar to nucleus transfer.

A more realistic outcome of blastomere separation would be the birth of twins, or possibly triplets, to a previously infertile couple. However, this should be no more objectionable than the natural creation of twins or triplets. It might be objected that blastomere separation makes it possible for twins to be born years apart. Although this would be a novel situation, it is not obvious that there is anything inherently wrong with it. If there is a long delay between births — say, twenty years — a possible objection is that the younger twin might prefer not to see what she will look like when she is older. However, such knowledge does not appear to be so dreadfully awful that we should discourage blastomere separation on its account. Moreover, if it were not for blastomere separation, a twin born years later would not exist. Thus, one could not reasonably claim that the second twin is *harmed* by blastomere separation — unless knowing what you will look like in the future is a fate worse than death!

Another possible objection is that blastomere separation might damage preembryos, resulting in birth defects. In reply, the technique has been used extensively in the cattle industry without increasing the incidence of birth defects. Nevertheless, the effect on human preembryos might be different. This concern could be addressed by carrying out chromosomal studies on human preembryos following blastomere separation, to see if there is an increased incidence of defects. If future evidence indicates that there is no increase in risk of birth injury, then clinical trials could be ethically justifiable, based on the potential to improve IVF success rates.

Disposition Following Divorce

When the dispute between Mary Sue and Junior Lewis Davis gained national attention, many IVF programs began requiring prefreezing agreements. As a result, divorce disputes in which there is no prefreezing agreement, as in the Davis case, have become infrequent. Despite this fact, the question of how to resolve divorce-related disputes over frozen preembryos continues to be important, for several reasons. First, prefreezing agreements are not a panacea, as illustrated by the divorce of Mary and Fred Wendel of Chagrin Falls, Ohio.[68] They had a prefreezing agreement stating that in the event of divorce, Mr. Wendel would be permitted to obtain or destroy the preembryos. However, after filing for divorce, Mrs. Wendel sought and obtained a restraining order to prevent her husband from disposing of their two preembryos, which were stored at the Cleveland Clinic Foundation. She argued that his obtaining them would eliminate her last and only chance for pregnancy and childbirth. Incidentally, the restraining order also prevented Mr. Wendel from obtaining their two Labrador retrievers and their season tickets to the Cleveland Browns!

Second, there are problems with the prefreezing agreements themselves. The terms of these agreements often are decided by the operators of the IVF programs, rather than the patients, and may reflect the values of the physicians rather than the gamete providers.[69] This is illustrated by an agreement document previously used at my own institution—a standardized form that was presented to all IVF patients. The problem was that it did not address all of the possible options; it did not allow the couple to express a preference that their preembryos be donated to other couples or a preference that they be used for research.

Several considerations support the view that infertile couples should not be required to sign prefreezing agreements before proceeding with IVF. One reason is that patients might not be able to predict accurately how they will feel about disposition of preembryos at a later time. In addition, there is an element of duress involved in requiring such agreements; often there is only one IVF program in a given locality, and patients who would prefer not to sign a prefreezing agreement might find it difficult to refuse. Thus, patients who are unsure concerning the disposition they would want might sometimes feel pressure to sign an agreement anyway.

When entered into under duress, such agreements should be legally voidable.[70] Whenever such agreements are *required* by an IVF program, it can be argued that they are potentially voidable on grounds of duress.

Although they should not be required, such agreements should be offered, and patients should have the option of entering into them or declining to do so. When such agreements are entered into free of duress, they should be regarded as legally enforceable. The ground for making them enforceable is that they are a more efficient method for resolving disputes than litigation. A couple should be free to revise their agreement at any time, provided they can mutually agree on the revisions.

The above discussion has several implications for health professionals who counsel patients about prefreezing agreements. It is apparent that careful and thorough counseling is needed. All of the possible uses of the preembryos should be identified. Patients should be advised that the passage of time might alter their feelings about disposition of frozen preembryos. They should be encouraged to recognize this and take it into account before entering into a prefreezing agreement. Also, flexibility should be permitted; although a standardized form might be used, additional provisions that tailor the agreement to the particular couple should be allowed.

When there is a dispute following divorce and either there is no prefreezing agreement or the agreement is legally voided because of duress, then an ethical basis is needed for deciding whose wishes should prevail. Typically, these disputes involve a conflict between freedom to procreate and freedom not to procreate. According to our ethical framework, one should not automatically seek a prioritizing in which one of these values always prevails over the other. Rather, there is a presumption that the prioritizing should take place in the context of specific cases, based on morally relevant casuistic factors that can vary from case to case. In these divorce disputes, the casuistic factors include the likelihood, degree, and reversibility of harm to the man and woman if their wishes do not prevail. Harms that can be caused by interfering with freedom not to procreate in this context include: the psychological harms involved in having a child but being unable to make rearing decisions; and financial burdens that might legally be imposed. Harms caused by interfering with freedom to procreate include the continuation of suffering experienced in being unable to have children. This suffering might be removed, however, if reproduction with another partner is feasible. Another casuistic factor is "sweat equity." Typically, in infertility treatment the woman is subjected to greater risks, pain, and inconvenience than the man. Fairness suggests that such differences in sweat equity should be considered in deciding whose wishes should prevail. Whether priority should be given to freedom to procreate or to freedom not to procreate depends on the casuistic factors present in a given case. A relatively strong argument for giving priority to freedom to procreate, for example, would be given in the following situation: the woman is infertile and wants to procreate with the preembryos; she has contributed a considerable amount of sweat equity; there is no likely alternative way for her to procreate; and there would be no legally required financial burdens on the man. In contrast, a relatively strong argument for giving priority to freedom not to procreate would exist in the following circumstances: the woman is infertile and wants to procreate with the preembryos; there is an alternative way for her to procreate, such as IVF with a new spouse; and she has contributed only a moderate amount of sweat equity, as might occur if there is oocyte donation rather than retrieval of her own oocytes. This method of reasoning illustrates the modified casuistic approach I defended in Chapter 4.[71]

Time Limits for Storage

Some ethics committee reports have recommended specific time limits for storage of frozen preembryos. For example, the Warnock report recommends ten years and claims that the need for a time limit is based on two considerations: the possibility of harmful effects of long storage on preembryos; and legal and ethical complications that might arise over disposal of preembryos whose parents have died or divorced.[72] However, these are not convincing reasons for time limits. Evidence based on animal preembryos suggests that there is no significant increase in birth defects based on long storage. In particular, studies of the effects of background radiation during storage failed to find any detrimental effects on preembryos exposed to the equivalent of about two thousand years of background radiation.[73] Moreover, the ethical and legal issues concerning death or divorce of progenitors can be handled by policies addressing those situations. If one progenitor dies, then the surviving progenitor should have full rights concerning disposition of preembryos. If both die without indicating their wishes concerning disposition, then one possible policy is to give decisional authority to the storage facility. Also, there are reasonable approaches for handling disputes following divorce, as discussed above. There are ways of dealing with these issues other than limiting the duration of storage.

Another view sometimes put forward is that there should be a time limit equal to the "reproductive life" of the progenitors. The problem with this view is the difficulty in defining a person's "reproductive life." There are several recent cases of women in their sixties giving birth following oocyte donation. Relatively older people are capable of raising children, and there is no clear place to draw a line representing the end of "reproductive life."[74]

Another possibility would be to limit storage to the lifetime of the progenitors. After both progenitors die, according to this view, preembryos would be removed from storage. Yet, even when both have died, it is not clear why it would always be necessary to remove preembryos from storage. If, for example, the progenitors had expressed a desire to turn the preembryos over to the storage facility, it might be more convenient for the facility to keep them in storage until a suitable time to use them for research or donation. The important thing is not that they be removed from storage but that there be a process for deciding the disposition of them.

It might be objected that an absence of time limits would make possible certain unusual family arrangements that could be harmful to the offspring. For example, children might be raised by elderly parents, twins might be gestated and reared years apart (assuming blastomere separation is used), or children might be gestated by their sisters or nieces. This objection makes the same mistake concerning the concept of harm that I discussed earlier. If it were not for the family arrangements in question, the children would not exist. The objection therefore states, in effect, that the children born into such nontraditional families are worse off than they would have been if they had not been conceived. However, it seems unreasonable to make this claim.

None of these arguments for limiting storage time is persuasive. If the progenitors want to keep their preembryos in storage for later possible use, are willing to pay the costs involved, and a storage facility is willing, then they should be permitted to do so.

7

New Genetics, New Decisions

An English couple who had a child with cystic fibrosis (CF) agreed to participate in a research study involving genetic testing of preembryos for CF, which is the most common lethal autosomal recessive disease among whites. They wanted to have another child but also wished to avoid a second child with CF. In addition, they wanted to avoid prenatal testing and abortion for CF. The woman, in her mid-thirties, received drugs to stimulate ovulation. Oocytes were retrieved and combined with her husband's sperm in vitro, and several of them became fertilized. When the fertilized ova grew into four- to eight-cell preembryos, a "biopsy" was performed on each one by holding it with a tiny suction tube and using another miniscule tube to extract a single cell. Segments of DNA in these cells were amplified and tested for the $\Delta F508$ defect, which was the cause of CF in the previous child. In two preembryos, both of the CF genes were defective, and these preembryos were rejected because a child produced would have the disease. Two other preembryos were selected for transfer to the woman's uterus; one was free of the defect in both genes and the other had the defect in one gene, making it a "carrier." The transfer resulted in pregnancy and the subsequent birth of a female infant. After birth, testing of the child revealed that both genes were normal — she was healthy and completely free of the CF defect.[1]

Such preimplantation testing has become possible because of impressive advances in the science and technology of gene mapping and sequencing. A growing number of gene defects that cause diseases have been identified. They include defects for sickle-cell anemia,[2] hemophilia,[3] Duchene muscular dystrophy,[4] neurofibromatosis type 1,[5] Huntington's disease,[6] cystic fibrosis,[7] and autosomal dominant polycystic kidney disease,[8] to mention a few. Tests that directly identify a number of these defects are now possible.[9] For other diseases, such as Marfan syndrome, family studies involving linkage analysis can detect the presence of defective genes.[10] Further progress will be fostered by the Human Genome Initiative, an international effort to analyze the structure of human DNA and identify the location of the estimated one hundred thousand human genes.[11] It is hoped that the information generated will enable us to understand and eventually treat many of the approximately five thousand genetic diseases that affect mankind. In the United States, the Human Genome Project is in the seventh year of a fifteen-year, three-billion-dollar program.[12]

As research continues, the number of available genetic tests will increase dramatically. Moreover, testing will be possible for new *categories* of conditions. One such category is susceptibilities to common diseases. There is evidence for genetic susceptibilities to diseases such as breast cancer,[13] colon cancer,[14] coronary artery disease,[15] insulin-dependent diabetes mellitus,[16] and bipolar affective disorder,[17] among others, and it is expected that genetic tests will become available to detect such susceptibilities. The term *susceptibility* is used because these diseases are considered to be *multifactorial*; the fact that an individual has an associated gene (or genes) does not necessarily mean that the disease will occur, because environmental factors might also contribute to disease onset. Thus, testing for susceptibilities would give information about an individual's *risks* of acquiring certain common diseases. Another category is adult-onset diseases. For example, direct tests are available to predict whether individuals will later be afflicted by Huntington's disease and autosomal dominant polycystic kidney disease. Also, there has been progress in the attempt to identify genes that cause Alzheimer's disease.[18] Further advances in predictive testing for a variety of adult-onset diseases can be expected.

In the future, these advances probably will become incorporated into routine health care. It seems likely that primary care physicians will inform patients of the availability of batteries of genetic tests for susceptibilities to common diseases.[19] Patients who consent will provide cell samples for such testing. With test results in hand, physicians can inform patients about multifactorial diseases for which they are at increased risk, such as colon cancer and heart disease. Patients can then be advised about changes in lifestyle that might help reduce their risks.

These rapid advances are raising a number of ethical questions in reproductive medicine. What genetic tests should be performed? Upon whom should they be performed? And in what situations? Moreover, research in gene therapy will increase our ability to alter the genetic make-up of individuals. We can envision a future in which it is possible to add and subtract selected DNA in germ cells and preembryos, raising additional questions. What genetic modifications, if any, should be performed? In what circumstances? These possibilities for testing and altering DNA open the door to designing human beings. Because these technologies can affect us profoundly, for better or worse, it is important for us to explore carefully the implications of these issues.

In this chapter, I shall focus on the following three areas: prenatal genetic testing for "minor diseases" and nondisease characteristics; testing of preembryos; and selection of gamete donors.[20] I have chosen these topics because they raise the issue of using genetics to modify man, and thus they confront what are potentially the most far-reaching issues raised by the new genetics.[21]

Prenatal Testing for "Minor Diseases" and Nondisease Characteristics

One implication of the new genetics is that we shall have an increased ability to test prenatally not only for serious diseases but also for relatively mild diseases, late-onset diseases, treatable diseases, elevated risks for common diseases, and eventually nondisease characteristics such as height and body build.[22] Prenatal testing for serious diseases followed by selective abortion has been regarded as ethically acceptable by the American public and the medical profession.[23] However, the new prenatal testing capabilities will create the possibility of selective abortion for relatively minor diseases as well as nondisease characteristics. To illustrate this issue, consider the following scenario, which is only a few years into the future. A pregnant woman with an elevated risk of carrying a fetus with Down syndrome is counseled by her obstetrician concerning prenatal testing for that condition. She agrees to testing and, in addition, states that because sample cells will be obtained for fetal tests, she would like the battery of tests for susceptibilities to common diseases carried out. Her physician asks why she is interested in having that information, and she says that if the fetus has any significant susceptibilities, she will have an abortion because she does not want her child to be at high risk for any of those diseases.[24]

The new genetics will make possible a number of "soft" reasons for abortion. Some might regard abortion for a detected susceptibility to disease to be ethically problematic, particularly if the test indicates a substantial probability of *not* getting the disease. Another type of situation involves a woman who would abort because of a fetal disease that is *treatable,* such as phenylketon-uria (PKU). Is it ethically justifiable to abort when the fetus's or infant's condition can be significantly controlled by treatment? What about an abortion performed because the fetus carries genes for an adult-onset disease? Presumably, there would be many years of good quality of life before onset of harmful symptoms. Another possibility would be selective abortion for nondisease characteristics, to enhance the quality of one's offspring. This might seem futuristic, but a goal of the Human Genome Project is to identify the complete nucleotide sequence of human DNA. Thus, data presumably will be available that can be used to look for correlations between genotype and phenotype for such attributes as intelligence and body build.

Readers who are skeptical that abortions would be sought for such reasons should consider the results of a survey by the New England Regional Genetics Group.[25] Couples were asked what types of genetic risks would lead them to terminate a pregnancy. One percent of couples said that if they had the information, they would consider terminating a pregnancy because the fetus was not the sex that they wanted. Six percent stated that they would abort a fetus that was susceptible to getting Alzheimer's disease in old age. Eleven percent said that they would abort a fetus that was susceptible to obesity. Thus, some people already embrace the idea of selecting the qualities of their offspring.

Abortions performed for these reasons following prenatal testing typically would involve presentient fetuses.[26] In Chapter 3, I argued that presentient fetuses have an intermediate moral status between embryos and late-gestation fetuses. Presentient fetuses should not be regarded as having a conferred right to life, but they should be accorded *some* degree of respect because of their partial similarity to paradigmatic persons. This status of partial respect might mean that some reasons for abortion are not morally weighty enough to justify it. The question before us is whether the "soft" reasons mentioned above are weighty enough to justify abortion of such fetuses.

From a clinical perspective, at least two questions can be distinguished: How should physicians respond to such requests, and which of these tests, if any, should routinely be offered to patients? I shall focus on the former question because I assume that the issue will first arise in clinical practice in the form of patient requests. The question takes two forms, depending on whether the physician is a geneticist or a primary care physician providing prenatal care. For geneticists, the question is whether the requested tests should be carried out; for primary care physicians, the issue is whether patients should be referred to geneticists, if any are available who are willing to perform the tests. The various views discussed below are relevant both to geneticists and primary care physicians.

MAIN VIEWS

Two views pertaining to this issue have been put forward. One was advocated by Angus Clarke, who proposed that prenatal testing should be restricted to the most severe disorders.[27] By this he means disorders involving either profound retardation, very severe physical handicaps, as in Duchene muscular dystrophy and Werdnig-Hoffman disease, or prolonged physical suffering, as in Huntington's disease and Fabry's disease. Clarke's view implies that physicians should refuse all requests for prenatal tests except those pertaining to the most severe disorders.

A second view attempts to draw a line somewhat closer to the mild end of the disease spectrum. Stephen G. Post, Jeffrey R. Botkin, and Peter Whitehouse have argued that patients' requests for prenatal tests should be honored except for diseases that are too minor.[28] They suggested that in deciding what is too minor, we should consider three dimensions of the severity of genetic diseases: the degree of harm to health if the disease occurs; the patient's age at onset of the disease; and the probability that genotype will influence phenotype. On their view, the strength of the argument for testing diminishes with decreasing degree of harm to health, increasing age of onset, and decreasing probability that phenotype will be affected. As an example, they suggest that familial Alzheimer's disease is not severe enough to justify prenatal testing followed by selective abortion, based on its late onset. Their approach is casuistic; in the context of each particular case, it attempts to weigh reproductive liberty against avoidance of abortion, using the three casuistic factors mentioned.

Let us consider what additional main views can be formulated concerning this issue. I believe that at least two can be identified. According to a third view, physicians should honor requests for prenatal tests for diseases and susceptibilities to diseases, but not requests pertaining to nondisease characteristics, such as gender, height, and intelligence. Although this specific view has not been advocated in the literature, the distinction between disease and nondisease has been put forward as a way to draw a line between interventions that are ethically permissible and those that are unacceptable, in the context of germ line gene therapy.[29] It is worth considering the application of this distinction to prenatal testing. According to a fourth view, all requests for prenatal tests should be honored, including those for minor diseases as well as nondisease characteristics. If these views were ordered in terms of the degree to which they withhold reproductive choices from pregnant women, the order would be as presented above, Clarke's view being the most restrictive.

With regard to these views, two issues can be distinguished: Which view is most justifiable ethically, and should any of these views be required or prohibited by law? I shall address both issues, beginning with the former. In assessing the ethical justifiability of these views, we should consider how they affect freedom not to procreate. In chapter two, I distinguished freedom not to procreate in the *strict* and *broad* senses. Specifically, freedom not to gestate in the strict sense includes freedom to decide to terminate a given pregnancy. If a woman's request for prenatal testing is refused, she still is free to decide to terminate the pregnancy. Thus, her freedom not to gestate in the strict sense has not been denied. However, her autonomy has been restrained because she has been denied information that, in light of her own values and goals, is highly relevant to her decision. We can say that she has encountered an obstacle to her freedom not to gestate in the broader sense, which includes freedom to *base* a decision to terminate pregnancy on the genetic characteristics of the fetus. In Chapter 2, I argued that freedom not to gestate in the strict sense should be respected because of its importance for self-determination. In applying that discussion to the present topic, we should ask whether freedom not to gestate in the broader sense also promotes self-determination. In assessing the four views identified above, we shall consider, among other things, the ways in which they promote or fail to promote self-determination.

PROS AND CONS

Let us consider the ethical pros and cons of these views. One of the problems with Clarke's view is that it fails to fulfill a central goal of prenatal testing and counseling: to enable couples to obtain information about childbearing risks and use that information to make informed voluntary choices, thereby promoting self-determination in reproductive decision making. This goal is widely recognized among geneticists as being important, and it was affirmed by the President's Commission in its report on genetic screening and counseling.[30] Clarke's approach cannot meet this goal because prenatal testing would be unavailable for those diseases that are not among the most severe according to his criteria. Examples of such diseases would include Down syndrome and hemophilia, neither of which typically involves profound retardation, severe physical handicap, or prolonged physical suffering. Nevertheless, they involve significant handicap or dysfunction, and pregnant women at risk of having a child with one of these conditions have an interest in being able to obtain appropriate prenatal tests, if wanted. This interest would be thwarted if Clarke's view were implemented.

A second, closely related, problem is that Clarke's view is inconsistent with the goal of nondirectiveness in counseling. Nondirectiveness refers to an approach in which genetic counselors attempt to avoid imposing their personal values upon the patient's decision. It involves, instead, helping patients make informed voluntary decisions based on their own values and goals. The main ethical justification for nondirectiveness is that it promotes the autonomy of couples making reproductive decisions.

Another reason supporting nondirectiveness is that it serves to dissociate genetic counselors from eugenics.[31] A brief historical digression will help explain this point. In the early 1900s, the eugenics movement gained momentum in the United States.[32] The American Eugenics Society came into being and soon became an influential voice in the eugenics movement. This organization advocated what it called the elimination of defectives, which was to be accomplished by segregating so-called defective individuals and by sterilization.[33] By 1937, thirty-one states had passed eugenic laws authorizing involuntary sterilizations of the mentally retarded, the mentally ill, epileptics, and habitual criminals, among others, based on the view that all of these conditions are inheritable. The total number of persons sterilized under these laws was over sixty-three thousand.[34] In Germany during World War II, the worst conceivable nightmares became reality, in the name of eugenics.[35] After World War II, the eugenics movement was widely, although not completely, rejected in the United States; involuntary sterilizations continued to be performed in some states into the 1960s.[36] During that decade, amniocentesis was beginning to be used as a method of obtaining fetal cells for karyotyping.[37] As prenatal diagnosis developed, it was recognized to be a technology that potentially could be used for eugenic purposes. It was perceived to be important to dissociate prenatal diagnosis from eugenics, and this provided one of the reasons why genetic counseling as a profession adopted nondirectiveness as its approach. Assuming that eugenics will continue to be an issue, the concern of genetic counselors to dissociate themselves from eugenics likely will remain valid.

Often it is pointed out that it is difficult if not impossible to be completely nondirective.[38] It is difficult to avoid sending messages, whether verbal or nonverbal, that reveal what the counselor believes should be done. However, even though it cannot be achieved perfectly, nondirectiveness is an important goal toward which to strive. Clarke's approach is based on the view that abortions for diseases other than the most severe ones are ethically unjustifiable, and in substituting this value judgment for that of the patient, his approach greatly deviates from nondirectiveness.

Let us consider the view of Post, Botkin, and Whitehouse. In support of their view, it might be argued that the prenatal detection of treatable diseases, late-onset diseases, or susceptibilities to diseases does not provide sufficiently weighty reasons to justify abortion, given that *some* respect should be accorded presentient fetuses. By adopting their view, physicians can avoid being an accessory to abortions for such minor reasons. However, the issue of non-directiveness again is relevant. In following the view of Post and colleagues, physicians substitute their judgments for those of patients concerning what is a serious enough disease or risk of disease to justify abortion. Even if this were to occur only for relatively minor diseases, nevertheless the goal of nondirectiveness would be put aside in those situations. Thus, the view of Post and colleagues poses a conflict between two ethical concerns: avoiding being an accessory to abortion for relatively minor reasons and providing nondirective counseling.

Several considerations support resolving this conflict in favor of nondirectiveness. First, the view of Post and colleagues underestimates the importance of preventing treatable or late-onset diseases in some families. For example, Louis J. Elsas described a case involving a mother of a three-year-old child with PKU who was pregnant again and requesting prenatal testing for PKU.[39] It is a disease that is treatable after birth by means of a special phenylalanine-free diet. The patient intended to have an abortion if genetic linkage analysis indicated that the fetus probably had PKU. Although the physician initially was hesitant to perform the test, the parents explained that care of their affected child involved significant financial and emotional costs. If they had two affected children, their emotional and economic resources for each child's care would be lessened. If they could choose, they would prefer not to have another child with PKU. Similar scenarios could be envisioned for late-onset disorders such as familial Alzheimer's disease. A couple might defend their request for prenatal testing as follows: "Grandfather suffered from Alzheimer's disease for years. His illness placed a heavy strain on our family, and we do not want the next generations of our family to go through the same ordeal." These examples are relevant to the concern that prevention of "minor" diseases is too trivial a reason to justify abortion. The examples suggest that, in some cases at least, this type of reason is not at all trivial.

Second, the view of Post and colleagues could inadvertently undermine the current professional consensus that nondirectiveness is important. In the future, genetic conditions will be detectable that have a range of severity. If physicians are encouraged to draw lines where they think diseases are "too minor," lines will be drawn in a wide variety of places. If Clarke's view is any indication, some physicians will draw the line at, or at least close to, very severe disorders, based on their personal values. Thus, the approach advocated by Post, Botkin, and Whitehouse threatens to to set aside nondirectiveness in favor of the freedom of physicians to draw the line where they wish. Whether a patient would be allowed to make her own reproductive decisions would depend on which physician provided her care. Therefore, the view in question should be rejected, since nondirectiveness is important for self-determination and no arguments have been given by Post, Botkin, and Whitehouse or others to justify such encroachments upon it.

Let us consider the view that all requests for prenatal testing should be honored. Although this view promotes freedom not to procreate in the broad sense more than the other three views, at least two types of objections can be made against it. The first focuses on the ethics of the abortions that would be involved. I shall argue that abortion for selection of nondisease characteristics, simply to satisfy the desires of parents, is not ethically justifiable. Consider abortion for selection of gender, for example, putting aside cases involving sex-linked diseases. Sex selection merely for parental preference seems to be a morally trivial reason for abortion, given that some degree of respect should be accorded to presentient fetuses. Perhaps it could be argued that in some cultures the child's gender is especially important, affecting a family's welfare because of economic and social institutions surrounding gender.[40] Even if such an argument would justify abortion for sex selection in some cultures — and I am not convinced that it would — it is not an acceptable argument as it applies to our culture. It is an argument that serves to perpetuate social attitudes and institutions that work to the disadvantage of women, and it should be rejected. Abortions for selection of other nondisease characteristics, such as superior height or above-average intelligence, also are morally unjustifiable because these reasons are not weighty enough, given that some respect should be given to the fetus.

Against these arguments, it could be pointed out that in the future very early selective abortions could be possible, particularly if it becomes possible routinely to sort fetal cells from maternal blood early in pregnancy and perform DNA analysis of the fetal cells.[41] It might be argued that the earlier the abortion, the less ethically problematic it is, and that very early abortions would be justifiable even if performed for selection of nondisease characteristics. In reply, the claim that reliable testing will be possible very early during gestation remains speculative. We simply do not know yet whether such an approach is feasible. Even if it turns out to be feasible, it might involve testing that is not much earlier in pregnancy than testing done by chorionic villus sampling. And even if very early selective abortion becomes possible, such abortions for enhancement still will be problematic because of arguments directed not against abortion but against the concept of designing our children.

This brings us to the second type of objection to the view in question. Several arguments can be stated against designing the characteristics of our children, based on possible adverse consequences. First, there is concern that parent-child relationships would be altered and that children might become more like "products."[42] Parents might then be less inclined to accept the strengths and weaknesses of their children. Such designing of offspring could erode the personal integrity and individuality of children and the adults they become. Altered parent-child relationships might have additional consequences; for example, less tolerance of children's imperfections might result in less compassion toward the handicapped. Also, there might be a greater tendency to blame parents for their children's imperfections. Children themselves might blame their parents, and this could disrupt some family relationships. Second, prenatal testing to enhance the characteristics of offspring likely would not be available to all, but would be skewed among different socioeconomic and ethnic groups. The reason is that the economically advantaged presumably would be better able to afford the costs of the tests and associated abortions. Because enhancement can increase a child's opportunities for improved socioeconomic status, unequal access to it would exacerbate current social and economic inequities.[43] Third, allowing parents to choose enhancement through prenatal testing and selective abortion would constitute a precedent in favor of positive eugenics. This could pave the way for other types of genetic engineering aimed at positive eugenics. The concern is that abuses might occur similar to those of previous eugenics programs, or that efforts will be made to redesign human nature, resulting in more harm than benefit.[44]

It should be acknowledged that designing our children could have positive consequences, as well. In some cases, enhancement might promote the happiness of parents and children and the quality of family life. Also, it has been pointed out that we do not have sufficient information fully to assess the risks and benefits of positive eugenics, and that we should not assume that positive eugenics is automatically wrong.[45] Admittedly, it is difficult to predict the long-term consequences of enhancement by means of prenatal testing and selective abortion. However, the arguments against designing our children raise significant enough concerns to suggest that we should not proceed with enhancement without a better understanding of where it might take us. These considerations provide added force to the argument that, for now at least, requests for prenatal testing and selective abortion for the "wrong" sex or hair color, or possession of merely average height or intelligence, should not be honored.

The above arguments support the view that physicians should honor requests for prenatal tests for diseases, including relatively minor diseases and susceptibilities to diseases, but not requests pertaining to nondisease characteristics. Concisely, the considerations favoring this view are the following: it preserves nondirectiveness better than the views of Clark and Post; it is easier to apply than the views of Clarke and Post because it is easier to distinguish disease from nondisease than to distinguish diseases that are "too minor" from those that are "not too minor"; given that early fetuses have limited moral standing, allowing an occasional abortion for "minor reasons" would seem to be acceptable if necessary to protect nondirectiveness; and we should be very cautious about pursuing selection for nondisease characteristics. This view is consistent with the idea that self-determination is important; freedom to abort for minor diseases helps prevent serious disruptions to a couple's self-determination, at least sometimes, as in the PKU case mentioned above. By contrast, abortion for sex selection or enhancement does not seem necessary to prevent severe disruptions to self-determination, in our culture at least.

This conclusion also is consistent with the method of assigning priorities defended in Chapter 4. I have argued, in effect, that the casuistic approach advocated by Post and colleagues is overridden by compelling reasons including the importance of nondirectiveness. This is an example of the modified casuistic approach I presented in Chapter 4 being preferable to the strict casuistic approach. Also, I have appealed to long-term consequences in rejecting the view that physicians should honor all requests for prenatal tests, further illustrating that the modified casuistic approach is capable of taking into account broad social implications.

OBJECTIONS AND REPLIES

It might be objected that the distinction between disease and nondisease traits is not always sharp. For example, a request for prenatal testing for morbid obesity might be motivated by a desire to avoid health problems related to obesity or, alternatively, to avoid an unattractive physique. Moreover, concerning such characteristics as low I.Q. and short stature, it is not always clear whether they are pathological or merely variations within normal limits.[46] In response, it must be acknowledged that the distinction has some gray areas. Nevertheless, the distinction is useful for contrasting many conditions. For example, PKU and cystic fibrosis clearly are diseases, whereas gender and above-average height clearly are not. Because the distinction usually is clear, in most cases it will be useful for guiding practice. Moreover, the distinction should be compared to the other proposals for line drawing, put forward by Clarke and by Post and colleagues. Certainly, there are no sharp lines for deciding which diseases are "most severe" or "too minor." An advantage of using the distinction between disease and nondisease is that in many cases the distinction is objective, based on pathophysiology. By contrast, deciding which diseases are too minor is more subjective. Thus, the former view seems to be less susceptible to wide variation in line drawing than the latter.

Another objection is that the view in question is susceptible to unreasonable requests by patients for testing. Let me respond by stating an important qualification to the view. Requests for tests for minor diseases sometimes will be unreasonable because they reflect a lack of knowledge by patients concerning such factors as the risks associated with testing, the probability that the fetus is affected, and the severity of the disease in question. In such cases the physician has a duty, in keeping with the goals of genetic counseling, to help the patient obtain a better understanding of such matters. It is to be hoped that, upon becoming better informed, the patient in many cases will reconsider the request.

An additional concern is that some geneticists would object on grounds of conscience to performing prenatal testing for disease susceptibilities, late-onset diseases, and relatively minor conditions, and some primary care physicians would conscientiously object to referring patients for such tests. Such conscientious refusals might be based on the degree of risk to the fetus in performing such tests. Even if such risks were removed by the development of noninvasive testing, conscientious objections might still be based on the degree of respect the physician believes should be given to fetal life. The view in question would honor conscientious objections by physicians, thereby showing respect for integrity, one of the virtues. However, such conscientious objectors should be aware that their refusals are inconsistent with nondirectiveness. Perhaps the best approach for geneticists in such cases is to refer the patient to another geneticist willing to carry out the test, if one is available. Similarly, primary care physicians should offer to arrange care by another physician.

Finally, it might be objected that refusing requests for tests for nondisease characteristics is a type of directiveness. Several views discussed above were rejected because of their directiveness, so why not reject the view in question for that reason? In response, I acknowledge that rejecting any request for testing involves directiveness. My task, therefore, is to defend the directiveness involved in the view in question. This brings us to some fundamental issues raised by advances in prenatal genetic testing: What should be the future purposes and role of medicine in this area? To what extent should physicians aim to satisfy the desires and demands of patients, and to what extent should they assert their own professional and personal values? I suggest that the directiveness involved in the view in question is defensible because it reflects a reasonable viewpoint concerning the purposes of reproductive genetic counseling. It proposes, in effect, that the purposes should focus on helping patients deal with diseases. This includes even minor diseases and susceptibilities to diseases. Within this domain, it states that physicians should strive to be nondirective. Tests for nondisease traits, however, would be regarded as outside the discipline of reproductive genetic counseling, and refusals to perform tests for nondisease characteristics would reflect practitioners' acceptance of this view concerning the purposes of the discipline.

This view draws upon an important conception of the role of the physician. Although physicians perform a variety of activities in their professional work, a central feature of the physician's role is helping patients and their families in matters of health and illness. The proposed conception of reproductive genetic counseling is based on this fundamental idea.

SHOULD THERE BE LEGAL RESTRICTIONS?

Should any of the views I have argued against be restricted legally? Let us begin by considering whether currently there are legal restrictions against them. In the United States there are legal barriers to the approach of providing prenatal testing only for the most severe diseases. Failure to inform pregnant women of the availability of tests for conditions such as Down syndrome, which presumably is not among the "most severe" as defined by Clarke, can result in malpractice lawsuits for wrongful birth.[47]

Such legal redress *should* be available, given the importance of helping pregnant women make informed, voluntary disease-related reproductive decisions. In theory, malpractice suits could also be brought against physicians who fail to honor requests for genetic tests for disease susceptibilities, late-onset diseases, and other "minor" diseases. However, such suits would succeed only if courts ruled that physicians have a legal duty to carry out such requests. Currently, no such legal duty has been established. With regard to the view that requests for testing for nondisease characteristics should be honored, at present there are no legal barriers.

The question, therefore, is whether additional legal restrictions should be imposed. One issue is whether physicians should have a legal duty to carry out requests for testing for susceptibilities to diseases, late-onset diseases, and diseases that involve relatively minor harms to health. Several considerations suggest that we should not establish a legal obligation on the part of physicians to honor such requests. One concern is that such a duty would be inconsistent with honoring conscientious refusals by physicians. It might be replied that the inconsistency can be avoided by having a legal duty *either* to carry out such requests *or* refer patients to physicians who will carry them out. However, this modified legal duty has shortcomings of its own. Recognizing such a duty would have the effect of conferring a significant degree of validation upon such patient requests. This might have the effect of significantly encouraging not only such requests for testing but also abortions for reasons having little moral weight. Moreover, creating such a duty might reinforce the desire for "perfect babies," thereby supporting attitudes in favor of enhancement. It is one thing to honor the occasional request for such testing; it is another thing to put legal policies in place that encourage such requests.

Another possible legal restriction would be to prohibit tests for nondisease characteristics. However, the fact that an action is ethically unjustifiable does not necessarily mean that it should be legally prohibited, given that such restrictions might interfere with important values to a degree not offset by the supposed benefits. In the present context, one such value is freedom not to procreate in the broad sense. Harms to future generations resulting from enhancement-related practices are somewhat speculative, as pointed out above. It has not been clearly demonstrated that such harms would be great enough to justify the intrusion upon reproductive freedom involved in a legal ban. Another argument against this legal restriction concerns a woman's right to choose abortion. Tests for enhancement purposes would be intertwined ethically with the abortion issue. At present, abortion before viability is legally available in the United States, regardless of the woman's reasons for seeking an abortion.[48] It seems inconsistent to permit abortions for all reasons but to make it illegal for a woman to obtain information relevant to certain reasons that are important to her.

The above considerations suggest that there should be no legal restrictions other than those already in place.

Genetic Testing of Preembryos

This chapter began with a case example involving preimplantation testing for CF. Preimplantation testing for serious genetic diseases like CF appears justifiable because it gives some couples the opportunity to have healthy offspring. As the number of available genetic tests increases, issues similar to those discussed above will arise for preimplantation testing: Would it be ethically justifiable to carry out requests to test preembryos for less severe conditions, such as treatable diseases, late-onset diseases, and susceptibilities to common diseases? What about testing and selecting preembryos for gender or enhancement? I argued above that physicians should not carry out requests for prenatal testing followed by abortion for nondisease characteristics. However, not transferring a preembryo to a woman's uterus is ethically less problematic than aborting a previable fetus, since there are differences in degree of similarity to the paradigm of descriptive persons, as discussed in Chapter 3. Thus, arguments against prenatal testing and abortion do not entail that preimplantation testing followed by discard of preembryos is wrong. It is necessary, therefore, to consider preimplantation testing separately.

TESTING FOR SUSCEPTIBILITIES AND LATE-ONSET DISEASES

Let us suppose that a couple undergoing in vitro fertilization (IVF) for infertility requests testing of their preembryos for disease susceptibilities or diseases that are minor, treatable, or late in onset, in order to select for replacement those preembryos that are most free of defects. Several considerations support the view that it is justifiable for physicians to carry out such requests. First, although such conditions generally are less serious, testing for them nevertheless would advance the goal of having healthy offspring. From the point of view of the child who would come into being, such selection is desirable because it helps avoid diseases. Second, carrying out requests for such tests would promote the couple's freedom to procreate in the broad sense and, to the extent that it avoids the birth of children with diseases, the couple's well-being. Moreover, because preembryos have only minimal moral standing, opposition to genetic testing of them based on the claim that they have serious moral standing is not justifiable.

It might be objected that because the degree of harm that would be prevented is less severe, the argument for carrying out such requests is not compelling. In reply, there can be significant burdens on families in some cases, as in the PKU example discussed above. Moreover, the burden on the one who suffers the disease can be very great for some late-onset conditions, such as Huntington's disease and autosomal dominant polycystic kidney disease.

Although preimplantation testing for relatively minor diseases, treatable diseases, late-onset diseases, and susceptibilities to diseases appears ethically justifiable, it is worth pointing out several issues that such testing would create. One issue arises because sometimes not many preembryos are available. This might occur because relatively few ova are recovered following ovarian hyperstimulation in a given case or because relatively few become fertilized in vitro. Moreover, although ova can be obtained from donors, the supply of such donor oocytes is limited at present.[49] When the number of preembryos is limited, discarding some because they carry genes for minor diseases or susceptibilities to diseases might reduce the probability that the woman would become pregnant. Thus, there would be a trade-off between having a child at all and avoiding diseases in the child. Such trade-offs likely would exist until such time, if ever, that success rates for IVF become very high or there is no scarcity of donated oocytes. One way in which some couples might deal with this trade-off would be to transfer the healthiest preembryos first. If these do not result in a pregnancy, then in subsequent cycles the couple might choose to transfer preembryos that carry genes for susceptibilities or minor diseases.

If a couple rejects one of their preembryos because it carries a susceptibility gene, then the disposition of that preembryo would raise a number of questions. Should donation of that preembryo to another infertile couple be considered? Would another couple want a preembryo that carries a gene for a susceptibility or late-onset disease? If so, would it be ethical to perform a uterine transfer using a preembryo with a known defect? Would it be better to use such preembryos for research rather than transfer them to a uterus? These issues would have to be addressed prior to preimplantation testing for susceptibility genes.

Another consideration arises when donated ova are used. An oocyte donor undergoes a certain amount of inconvenience and risk, and she might object to preembryos being discarded for what might be perceived as minor reasons. This raises the question of whether the donor should be told that preembryos might be rejected for such reasons. For some donors, such information might be material to the decision to donate. Therefore, it would be appropriate to reveal this information before donation.

TESTING FOR NONDISEASE CHARACTERISTICS

Genetic testing of preembryos gives rise to the possibility of testing for nondisease characteristics such as intelligence and body build. Preembryos carrying superior genes for these characteristics could be selected for replacement to the woman's uterus. Several considerations would support such testing. First, having a child with superior characteristics likely will promote the happiness of the parents. Second, from the offspring's point of view such selection is desirable because it is likely to give the child qualities that would be advantageous. However, in opposition to such selection, one can put forward the same arguments against designing our children discussed above. As I indicated earlier, the lessons of history suggest that we should proceed cautiously in this area. Also, the concerns about social inequities and harmful alterations in parent-child relationships are again pertinent. The arguments against designing our children support the conclusion that physicians should not honor requests by patients for preimplantation testing for enhancement. Again, I am not suggesting that positive eugenics could never be justifiable. Rather, I am suggesting that we would need a greater degree of confidence that the benefits would outweigh the harms before we would be ethically justified in proceeding.

However, it does not follow that preimplantation testing for enhancement should be legally forbidden. As I argued before, the fact that an activity raises ethical concerns does not necessarily mean that it should be prohibited, especially when the concerns are somewhat speculative. Given the uncertainty about whether enhancement would result in social harms, it is difficult to justify the intrusion into reproductive freedom in the broad sense that would be involved in a legal ban.

SEX SELECTION

What about preimplantation testing for sex selection? Again, I wish to focus on cases involving parental preference for a particular gender, rather than prevention of sex-linked diseases. Several arguments can be put forward against this method of gender selection. First, concerns have been raised that sex selection would lead to adverse social consequences due to an unbalanced sex ratio.[50] Second, it has been argued that sex selection is inherently wrong because it is a form of sexism.[51] Third, it has been argued that sex selection sets a precedent for positive eugenics.[52]

With regard to the first argument, it is likely that testing of preembryos would occur only in a small percentage of pregnancies. Such requests might be made by infertile or fertile couples, but in either case such testing typically would follow IVF. Infertile couples undergoing IVF comprise only a small percentage of all pregnancies. Fertile couples desiring sex selection might consider preimplantation testing, but the number actually requesting it would likely be small, due to several factors: the high cost of IVF; the need to administer superovulatory drugs that can have adverse side-effects; and the need to undergo an oocyte recovery procedure. Because only a small percentage of couples would seek preimplantation testing for sex selection, the impact on the sex ratio likely would be minimal. With regard to the second argument, although sex selection can be motivated by sexist attitudes, it need not be.[53] For example, a desire to have one child of each sex does not appear to be sexist. One might even have no preference concerning gender of the firstborn, thereby avoiding the sexism involved in wanting a male first.

The concern about positive eugenics is more difficult to overcome. It should be noted that sex selection is not itself a form of enhancement. To claim otherwise is to imply that one gender is superior to the other. However, it is clear that in our male-dominated society, being male confers advantages upon a person. The problem is that sex selection can set a precedent for positive eugenics because it can be described as selecting characteristics that confer advantages upon the offspring. Thus, the arguments given above against preimplantation selection for enhancement based on a rejection of eugenics also apply to preimplantation sex selection. I conclude that we should not encourage preimplantation sex selection at this time because of the concern about positive eugenics. Physicians should not carry out requests for gender selection based merely on parental preferences. However, as argued above concerning preimplantation selection for enhancement, preimplantation selection for gender should not be legally forbidden.

Selection of Gamete Donors

Donor insemination (DI) has been widely used in the United States for a number of years as a way of responding to male-factor infertility or, in some cases, to avoid transmission of genetic diseases. More recently, oocyte donation has been used successfully for infertile women who no longer can produce oocytes or who have difficulty becoming pregnant through IVF using their own oocytes. When a third-party donor is involved in the reproductive process, several ways of selecting the genetic characteristics of offspring become possible, in addition to those discussed above. These include testing donors for susceptibility genes and selecting donors to enhance the characteristics of offspring. To discuss the issues raised by these possibilities, it will be helpful to begin by briefly considering current practices concerning genetic screening in gamete donation.

Most discussions of genetic screening in gamete donation have focused on sperm donation, since it has been practiced longer than oocyte donation. I shall use the term *genetic screening* to refer to taking a genetic history and carrying out appropriate genetic tests. In 1979, a survey of physicians providing DI for male-factor infertility revealed that genetic screening of semen donors was inadequate.[54] Many of the physicians were not knowledgeable about genetics, and genetic history-taking often was cursory or omitted altogether. Following this report, a number of commentators agreed that there was a need for better genetic screening.[55] This raised the issue of what should be involved in such screening. In 1981, Timmons and colleagues proposed guidelines for genetic screening of sperm donors, emphasizing the need to obtain a genetic history from both the sperm donor and the female recipient.[56] At about the same time, Fraser and Forse[57] also proposed a set of guidelines, and other authors[58] soon followed with guidelines of their own. In 1993, guidelines were put forward by the American Fertility Society, now named the American Society for Reproductive Medicine (ASRM), that apply to both sperm and oocyte donation.[59] The ASRM guidelines recommend excluding donors with any of the following conditions: a major Mendelian disorder; a major multifactorial or polygenic malformation; a familial disease with a major genetic component; a chromosomal rearrangement; carrier state for an autosomal recessive gene known to be prevalent in the donor's ethnic background and for which carrier status can be detected; or advanced age (thirty-five or older for females, forty or older for males). Also, the ASRM guidelines propose that donors be rejected if they have a first-degree relative (parents or offspring) with any of the following: a major multifactorial or polygenic disorder; a major autosomal dominant or X-linked disorder with late age of onset or reduced penetrance; an autosomal recessive disorder, if the disorder has a high frequency in the population and the donor's gametes will be used on many occasions; or a chromosomal abnormality, unless the donor has a normal karyotype. The ASRM guidelines state that the same genetic screening carried out on sperm donors should be offered to the female recipients of donated sperm. However, in addressing oocyte donation, the guidelines fail to state that genetic screening should be offered to the male partner who provides the sperm. This seems to be an oversight; to help avoid genetic disease in the offspring, the male partner also should be offered screening.[60]

As the number of available genetic tests increases, certain changes in these guidelines might become appropriate. One type of change is that testing will be available in lieu of automatically excluding certain potential donors. For example, current guidelines recommend rejecting donors who have first-degree relatives with major autosomal dominant disorders with late age of onset, such as adult-onset polycystic kidney disease. In the future, we will be able to accept such donors if they have been tested and found to be free of the gene defect. Similarly, testing might be considered instead of automatic exclusion when the donor has a first-degree relative with a major x-linked disorder with late age of onset or reduced penetrance, or an autosomal recessive disorder, if the disorder has a high frequency in the population. Any genetic testing of gamete donors, of course, should be performed only if informed consent is given.

TESTING DONORS FOR SUSCEPTIBILITY GENES

As tests for susceptibility genes become available, one issue that will arise is whether gamete donors should be tested for susceptibilities to common diseases such as colon cancer, breast cancer, and coronary artery disease. It will be possible to select the genetic characteristics of offspring, to some extent, by rejecting donors with susceptibility genes.

Rejecting donors who have susceptibility genes appears to be ethically justifiable, based on several considerations. First, from the offspring's point of view, it is desirable to avoid serious diseases, regardless of whether their onset is early or late. Second, freedom not to procreate in the broad sense includes freedom to avoid procreation with a donor who has an undesirable genetic make-up. Rejection of a donor would be especially justifiable when necessary to promote the self-determination of the recipient couple, as when the child would have a significant chance of developing a serious early-onset disease.

According to the current ASRM guidelines, potential donors who have a first-degree relative with a common familial disease would be rejected.[61] A genetic history often would identify donors at risk of transmitting such diseases. In the future, as tests for susceptibility genes become available and costs decrease, testing donors at risk might become preferable to outright rejection, at least for some donors. In particular, it might be preferable in oocyte donation, if the supply of oocytes continues to be scarce. If the particular oocyte donor is free of the defect in question, then her oocytes can be used even though the disease runs in her family. Eventually, it might become reasonable to screen prospective donors routinely for certain familial diseases even when there is a negative family history, for several reasons. First, some familial diseases might have reduced penetrance or variable expressivity, and the donor might report a negative history even though the defective gene is carried in the donor's family. Second, a few donors might simply not be well informed concerning the health status of family members.

For some susceptibility genes, the severity of the disease and likelihood that the child would acquire the disease might be relatively low. This raises the question concerning what degree of severity and likelihood would be required to justify routinely performing a test on potential donors, assuming it has a low cost, is reliable, and informed consent is given. One might answer by using as a benchmark those diseases that have a high enough severity and likelihood of occurrence that currently we routinely test for them, at least in defined populations. One example is sickle-cell anemia, which has a carrier frequency of one in ten to twelve among African-Americans. Similarly, Tay-Sachs disease has a carrier frequency of one in thirty among Ashkenazi Jews. Both are autosomal recessive, so there is a 25 percent chance of transmitting the disease if both parents are carriers. A strong argument could be made for routinely testing for common familial diseases that have a severity and likelihood of occurrence in a given population that are comparable to, or higher than, that of sickle-cell anemia among African-Americans or Tay-Sachs disease in Ashkenazi Jews. An example might be hereditary nonpolyposis colorectal cancer, for which it is estimated that one in two hundred Americans carry the defective gene.[62] An individual who carries the gene is estimated to have a 70 to 90 percent chance of getting colon cancer.[63] Thus, it is a serious disease with a likelihood of occurrence in the general population that is comparable to that of sickle-cell anemia among Ashkenazi Jews. Currently, the cost of testing for the gene for hereditary nonpolyposis colorectal cancer is approximately one thousand dollars.[64] Thus, at present it would be more reasonable simply to reject donors at risk than to incur the expense of testing, but when the cost becomes low this is likely to change.

Other susceptibility genes might be very rare, and if tests for them were available, they need not routinely be carried out. Between the rare diseases and those for which routine screening clearly should be performed there will be a continuum in terms of severity and likelihood of occurrence. There will be a gray area involving familial diseases with severity and likelihood of occurrence somewhat lower than those for which routine screening clearly is warranted. One approach to such diseases would be to inform the recipient and her male partner of the availability of tests but not routinely to perform or recommend them.

Guidelines in the future, therefore, might involve several categories of tests. For some tests — those involving diseases with relatively high severity or likelihood of occurrence — the physician would *recommend* that the tests be carried out. For other tests, the physician would discuss the availability of the test but encourage the infertile couple to make their own decision. The question of what tests should be included in these categories is best decided by an interdisciplinary group. The Ethics Committee of the ASRM has assumed a leadership role in issuing its previous guidelines, and it is an example of an appropriate body to address these questions as new tests arise.[65]

SELECTION OF GAMETE DONORS TO ENHANCE THE
QUALITY OF OFFSPRING

Another issue is whether gamete donors should be selected to enhance the characteristics of offspring. Recipients might want to select donors who are intelligent, beautiful, or have a good physique. Is such selection ethically justifiable?

Because DI has been a relatively widespread practice in the United States for several decades, it will be helpful to begin by considering the extent to which selection for superior characteristics has been part of the practice of sperm donation. In 1988, the Office of Technology Assessment published the results of a survey of a national sample of sperm banks and physicians who provide artificial insemination.[66] Several survey questions asked about matching the characteristics of the sperm donor to those of the social father. According to an estimate based on a weighted sample of 367 physicians, 72 percent of physicians who provided artificial insemination were willing to "select donor characteristics to recipient specifications." Among those so willing, 90 percent would match for height, 82 percent for body type, 66 percent for educational attainment, 57 percent for I.Q., and 45 percent for special abilities, such as athletic skills. All fifteen sperm banks surveyed permitted recipients or their physicians to specify donor traits. Among the fifteen sperm banks, fourteen would match for height, fourteen for body type, eleven for special abilities, eleven for educational attainment, and seven for I.Q. One sperm bank, the Repository for Germinal Choice, specializes in semen samples from donors who are highly intelligent and accomplished.[67]

Thus, a substantial percentage of physicians who provide artificial insemination and sperm banks are willing to participate in selection that could be described as enhancement. However, this selection purportedly is carried out to match characteristics of social father and donor. Given the widespread tendency in DI to maintain secrecy concerning the offspring's genetic origins,[68] it is reasonable to assume that social fathers often desire matching because it helps promote secrecy. It is unclear to what extent recipients' specification of donor characteristics is motivated by the desire for enhancement as opposed to secrecy. In selecting mates, of course, people often consider what the offspring would be like. Sometimes mates are chosen, in part, because it seems likely that they will transmit desirable characteristics. Clearly, such selection constitutes a method of enhancing the quality of offspring. It seems reasonable to conclude, therefore, that even when selection of sperm donors is motivated by secrecy, it sometimes indirectly serves enhancement because it matches a male partner who was himself selected in part because of enhancement considerations.

It is worth noting that, according to the survey, 20 percent of physicians who provided DI were unwilling to select donor characteristics based on the recipient's specifications.[69] Also, among the 72 percent who were willing to do so, a number were unwilling to fulfill certain types of specifications. Specifically, 29 percent would not select for educational attainment, 37 percent were unwilling to select for I.Q., and 50 percent would not select for special abilities. Also, most of the respondents from the fifteen sperm banks were opposed to the type of semen banking performed by the Repository for Germinal Choice.[70] Thus, although some selection for enhancement seems to occur, there is a lack of consensus among professionals involved in DI that enhancement is acceptable.

Because oocyte donation is relatively new, there is little data on selection of oocyte donors. Published reports suggest that selection of donors based on education[71] or other characteristics requested by recipients[72] takes place to some extent. However, the relatively small number of oocyte donors, compared to sperm donors, may limit the extent to which selection for enhancement occurs at present. In the future, technical advances such as primordial follicle donation could increase the supply of oocytes,[73] and this would make selection for enhancement more feasible.

Although I have argued against prenatal and preimplantation testing for enhancement, several considerations suggest that selecting gamete donors for enhancement is ethically acceptable. First, as mentioned above, selection for offspring characteristics often is a consideration in choosing mates, and such selection seems to be ethically justifiable. Since we value reproductive freedom, we should value the freedom of individuals to select mates based on their personal preferences, including preferences that take into account the possible characteristics of offspring. If it is ethically permissible to take such considerations into account in selecting mates, then it also seems permissible to take them into account in selecting gamete donors. Both types of situations involve reproductive freedom in choosing a genetic parent for one's offspring. Second, from the point of view of the offspring's interests, selection of oocyte and sperm donors with superior characteristics is desirable because it is likely to give the offspring qualities that would be advantageous. Third, having a child with superior characteristics is likely to promote the happiness of the parents.

On the other hand, the argument that we should avoid positive eugenics is again applicable. Enhancement through selection of gamete donors might set a precedent for positive eugenics. However, a response can be made to this argument. There are ways of setting precedents *against* positive eugenics other than preventing selection of gamete donors. For example, a policy that discourages prenatal testing and abortion for enhancement purposes, as defended above, would constitute such a precedent. Similarly, a policy that discourages testing preembryos for enhancement would serve as a precedent. Assuming that we should take a stand against positive eugenics, several considerations suggest that selection of gamete donors is not the best place to do it. First, selection of gamete donors for enhancement purposes is similar to the justifiable and deeply entrenched practice of selecting mates partly on the basis of enhancement considerations. As stated above, it is difficult to argue that the latter is justifiable but the former is not. Second, matching gamete donors to social parents seems justifiable, independently of the pros and cons of maintaining secrecy about the child's genetic origins. Even parents who would not be secretive about the child's origins might want the child to resemble the social parents in certain ways. Race and ethnic background are obvious examples. Moreover, it is difficult to permit matching without enhancement being implicated. For example, tall parents might prefer tall children, and highly intelligent parents might prefer intelligent children. These arguments support the view that selection of gamete donors for enhancement is ethically acceptable, although abortion as well as testing preembryos for enhancement are not.

8

Fetal Anomalies
Treatment and Abortion Decisions

Technological advances such as ultrasonography and chorionic villus sampling have increased the ability of obstetricians to detect fetal anomalies in utero, and future advances in genetic testing promise to increase this ability further. When anomalies are detected before viability, abortion is legally available in the United States based on the 1973 Supreme Court decision in *Roe v. Wade*.[1] However, sometimes anomalies are not diagnosed until later in gestation, and even when they are detected before viability, the woman sometimes chooses to continue the pregnancy. When abortion is not performed, questions arise concerning treatment during pregnancy. New techniques have improved the obstetrician's ability to intervene when medical conditions occur that are potentially harmful to the viable fetus. Examples include use of tocolytic drugs to halt premature labor, emergency cesarean section when fetal monitoring detects serious problems, and experimental fetal therapy in some situations.[2] The capability of intervening in these ways raises questions concerning how aggressively the pregnant woman and obstetrician should strive to promote fetal well-being when anomalies are present.

An illustration is provided by the following case, which occurred at my institution. A twenty-four-year-old married woman was a patient at the university obstetrical service. Ultrasound examinations revealed that her fetus had hydrocephalus—an excessive accumulation of cerebrospinal fluid in the brain—as well as spina bifida in the lumbar region of the back. The hydrocephalus could cause brain damage and mental retardation if the infant survived, and the spina bifida could cause paralysis of the legs and incontinence of bowel or bladder. At thirty-five weeks' gestational age, another ultrasound revealed that the fluid build-up was causing the fetal head to be larger than normal, and this raised several questions. If the fetus were carried to term but its head were too large to pass through the birth canal, would it be ethical for the physician to reduce the head size by means of cephalocentesis (draining cerebrospinal fluid from the cranium), given that this procedure usually causes fetal death? Alternatively, should the physician recommend cesarean section to avoid having to drain the fetal head for vaginal delivery? Which method of delivery should be used?[3]

This chapter explores issues raised by this and other cases involving fetal anomalies. To limit the length of discussion, I focus mainly on the question of what recommendations, if any, the physician should make to the pregnant woman in these types of cases. Before we attempt to answer this question, we need to consider three main ways in which the ethical framework developed in Part 1 can be brought to bear on it.

First, the framework helps us identify relevant ethical values. It maintains that there is a plurality of values relevant to decisions in bioethics, and it requires us to take into consideration all values relevant to a given issue. Several values are especially pertinent to decisions during pregnancy, and it is worthwhile to identify them explicitly. One is the principle of autonomy, according to which the informed and well-considered choices of mentally competent persons should be respected. It is the basis of the pregnant woman's right to make decisions concerning abortion and treatment during pregnancy. The principle of autonomy also applies to physicians and entails, among other things, that there should be respect for the physician's desire to avoid unethical or illegal actions and to practice in accordance with reasonable professional standards.

Another relevant value is the principle of beneficence, which holds that we should promote the well-being of individuals and avoid harming them.[4] This principle applies to all parties involved in the situations in question. The well-being of the pregnant woman is an important consideration, and the physician has obligations to preserve and promote the woman's health and avoid causing harm to her. Similarly, the well-being of the fetus is relevant; when the fetus has a significant conferred moral standing, the pregnant woman and physician have obligations to act beneficently toward the fetus. Even when the fetus does not have a significant conferred moral standing but the woman intends to carry it to term, she and the physician have obligations to promote the fetus's well-being, based on a concern for the future child.

Moreover, it will prove helpful to distinguish two duties that the physician has to act beneficently toward the fetus. The physician can have a duty *to the fetus* to act beneficently toward it and also can have a distinct duty *to the pregnant woman* to act beneficently toward her fetus. The duty to the fetus rests on the fetus's moral standing. To see this, let us suppose that a particular fetus should be regarded as having a conferred moral status that is very close in strength to that of normative personhood. In that event, the argument for respecting the well-being of the fetus would be relatively strong. It would be plausible to say that others have a duty to that fetus to avoid causing it harm, although that duty might be slightly less strong than the duty to avoid harming individuals who have full normative personhood status. This would be a duty owed to the fetus itself because of its moral standing. By contrast, a duty to the pregnant woman to act beneficently toward her fetus would be based on respect for *her* as a person. Respect for her autonomy requires protecting the well-being of her fetus, if that is her wish. Similarly, respect for her well-being requires protecting the well-being of her fetus, if it is reasonable to believe that failing to do so would diminish the pregnant woman's well-being. In assessing whether the physician should act beneficently toward the fetus, it is necessary to consider both of these duties. In some cases, the physician might have only a weak duty to the fetus but a relatively strong duty to the woman. An example would arise when there is little that can be done to benefit a fetus with severe anomalies, but the woman autonomously insists on doing everything possible. In other cases, the physician could have relatively strong duties both to the fetus and woman to act beneficently toward the fetus.

In addition, the well-being of the physician is important. Physician well-being would be especially relevant, for example, when contemplated actions by the physician would involve risks of legal liability or criminal prosecution. This supports the view that there are limits to the legal risks physicians can reasonably be expected to take for the sake of patients.

A third value is the principle of avoiding killing, which is relevant because procedures that can cause fetal death are sometimes considered; namely, abortion as well as cephalocentesis to deliver a fetus with hydrocephalus. This principle expresses a social norm that it is wrong to take the lives of innocent persons.[5] In addition to this general principle against killing, physicians have a special role responsibility to respect and preserve the lives of patients.[6] This responsibility gives added seriousness to situations in which killing by physicians is being contemplated. As before, it will be helpful to distinguish between two duties that the physician can have to avoid killing the fetus. The physician can have a duty *to the fetus* to avoid killing it and a duty *to the pregnant woman* to avoid killing her fetus. Again, a duty to the fetus would rest on the fetus's moral standing and a duty to the pregnant woman would rest on respect for her as a person.[7]

A second way in which the ethical framework bears on these questions concerns the moral status of fetuses that have serious anomalies. In Chapter 3, I argued that the more similar a fetus is to the paradigm of descriptive persons, the stronger the argument for conferred moral standing. Several morally relevant similarities to persons in the descriptive sense were identified: the potential to *cause* self-consciousness; the potential to *become* self-conscious; similarity in appearance to the paradigm; viability; sentience; having been *born*; and a social role. Based on these similarities, I argued that it is justifiable to confer normative personhood status upon normal newborn infants. Also, I pointed out that normal fetuses that are relatively advanced in development are close in similarity to the paradigm, and that consequentialist considerations support conferring upon them a moral status that is close to, although slightly less than, that of newborns. However, in the present chapter we shall see that some extremely severe anomalies have the effect of diminishing the degree of similarity a fetus has to the paradigm. For example, some anomalies deprive fetuses of sentience or the potential for self-consciousness even though they are relatively advanced in gestation. A diminished similarity to the paradigm would justify a diminished moral standing for the fetus.

A diminished fetal moral status would have implications for the weight of the ethical values that are relevant to the fetus. In particular, the weight that should be given to the physician's duty to the fetus to act beneficently toward it depends on its moral standing.[8] If a given fetus has a moral standing that is close to normative personhood, then the physician has a relatively strong duty to the fetus to act beneficently toward it. On the other hand, if there is diminished moral standing due to extremely severe anomalies, then the strength of the physician's duty to the fetus to act beneficently is lessened. This does not necessarily mean, however, that there is *no* duty to such a fetus to act beneficently toward it or that the physician's duty to the pregnant woman to act beneficently toward her fetus is lessened.

Similarly, the moral standing of the fetus has implications for the strength of the duty to the fetus to avoid killing it. If a given fetus has a moral standing that is close to normative personhood, then the physician has a relatively strong duty to the fetus to avoid killing it. On the other hand, if the fetus has diminished moral standing, then the strength of the physician's duty to the fetus to avoid killing it is lessened.[9] Again, this does not mean that the physician has no duty to the fetus to avoid killing it or that the physician's duty to the pregnant woman to avoid killing the fetus is diminished.

A third way in which the framework is relevant to these cases concerns the assigning of priorities to conflicting ethical values. In Chapter 4, I argued for a casuistic approach to weighing conflicting values. An important aspect of that approach is the identification of casuistic factors. The degree to which each of these factors is a feature of a case can vary from one case to the next. The assigning of priorities to conflicting values is based on the degree to which the various factors are present in the case at hand. More will be said about casuistic factors in the sections below that deal with specific types of fetal anomalies.

Options for Decision Making

The physician has an obligation, based on respect for the pregnant woman's autonomy, to help her make informed decisions concerning medical care during pregnancy. When fetal anomalies are detected, this obligation requires the physician to discuss the options concerning medical management. There seem to be four main approaches to medical management in these circumstances. One option is abortion, which legally is available in all states prior to viability. However, access to abortion before viability is limited because many localities have no providers of abortion services. After viability, the availability of legal abortion is even more limited. According to one study of abortion law, abortion for any reason after viability is legal only in New Jersey, Ohio, and Oregon.[10] In addition, postviability abortion when the fetus has severe anomalies is legal in Colorado, Kansas, New Mexico, and Texas, but in these states it sometimes is unclear how serious the anomaly must be for abortion to be legal.[11] In all other states, abortion after viability is lawful only to preserve the life or health of the pregnant woman.[12] To promote informed consent, the physician should inform the woman concerning the legal availability of abortion in her locality before and after viability.[13]

A second option is to continue the pregnancy with management aimed at optimizing maternal well-being. Conflicts between maternal and fetal well-being would be resolved by giving priority to maternal interests. This *nonaggressive* approach avoids procedures involving increased maternal risks, such as tocolysis or cesarean delivery for fetal indications. The third approach is to continue the pregnancy and attempt to optimize the welfare of the fetus. Conflicts between fetal and maternal well-being would be resolved by giving priority to fetal interests. This *aggressive* approach uses medical and surgical procedures indicated for fetal well-being even though increased risks would be involved for the woman. A fourth option continues the pregnancy using an intermediate approach that balances maternal and fetal interests. This *balancing* would permit exposure of the woman to risks for the sake of the fetus in some, but not all, situations. In this approach, the degree of risk to the woman posed by a procedure and the likelihood of benefit to the fetus are among the casuistic factors that would be considered in making decisions in specific circumstances. Discussing these four options is an appropriate way for the physician to begin a dialogue with the pregnant woman aimed at helping her make informed decisions.

Prior to viability, usually there are few, if any, possible invasive therapeutic interventions for the sake of the fetus. Experimental fetal therapy might be possible in certain situations, but such therapy typically is available only at a small number of research centers.[14] Thus, except for unusual cases involving experimental therapy, there generally is no necessity to implement choices among the aggressive, nonaggressive, and balancing approaches prior to viability, although it might often be appropriate to discuss these options before viability, if doing so would help prepare the pregnant woman for decisions later in pregnancy.[15] Rather, prior to viability the main focus of discussion of the options typically is on a decision concerning abortion. The physician should discuss the abortion option in a nondirective manner, unless continuing the pregnancy poses a serious risk to the health or life of the woman. If such risks to the woman exist, then it is ethically justifiable for the physician to recommend abortion. Several considerations support directive counseling in this relatively uncommon type of situation. First, the woman presumably has entered the physician-patient relationship, in part, to seek help from the physician in promoting her own health. Given this context, recommendations typically are part of what patients want and expect, and it seems reasonable to say that the physician has an obligation to make recommendations, based on sound medical judgment, concerning the woman's health. Second, when continuing the pregnancy poses grave risks to the life of the woman, an effective way for the physician to communicate the seriousness of these risks, so as to avoid misunderstanding, is to include in the discussion a recommendation of pregnancy termination.

The moral justification of abortion prior to viability is based on considerations of the moral status of the fetus and the autonomy and well-being of the pregnant woman. As I argued in Chapter 3, viability itself is not a criterion of personhood. What is relevant is the degree of similarity of the fetus to the paradigm of descriptive persons. Because this similarity is, at best, only moderate for the previable fetus, normative personhood status is not justifiable. The fetus has a diminished moral standing compared to descriptive persons and, as I argued above, the principle of avoiding killing has diminished force.

In Chapter 2, I discussed the importance of autonomy, or self-determination, particularly in regard to women, for whom self-determination is especially important for the gaining of social, political, and economic equality. These considerations support the view that the autonomy of the woman outweighs the moral status of the previable fetus. Even if the fetus is medically normal, the woman's autonomy overrides during this period of gestation. If the fetus has anomalies that further diminish the similarity with the paradigm, that strengthens the argument for the ethical permissibility of abortion.

Abortion after Twenty-four Weeks

In most states, abortion after viability is illegal except when necessary to protect the life or health of the pregnant woman. To have a better understanding of when abortion is not legally an option, it is necessary to consider the specifics of the Supreme Court rulings concerning viability. In *Roe v. Wade,* the Court stated that the fetus becomes viable when it is "potentially able to live outside the mother's womb, albeit with artificial aid."[16] It also stated that a viable fetus "presumably has the capability of meaningful life outside the mother's womb."[17] In *Colautti v. Franklin,* the Court elaborated upon these comments, stating that by "meaningful life" it had meant "not merely momentary survival."[18] In *Planned Parenthood of Central Missouri v. Danforth,* the Court ruled that states may not draw a line defining viability at any particular gestational age or birth weight. Rather, the determination of viability is left to the judgment of the physician in each individual case. In the words of the Court: "The time when viability is achieved may vary with each pregnancy, and the determination of whether a particular fetus is viable is, and must be, a matter for the judgment of the responsible attending physician."[19]

Further comment on the definition was provided in *Colautti,* where the court stated: "Viability is reached when, in the judgment of the attending physician on the particular facts before him, there is a reasonable likelihood of the fetus [sic] sustained survival outside the womb, with or without artificial support."[20] The Court used the term "sustained survival," but it has never offered clarification concerning the length of time an infant must be kept alive in order to achieve "sustained survival." Although the Court stated that it must be more than merely momentary survival, this leaves considerable room for interpretation. Also, the Court has never clarified what it meant in stating that there must be a "reasonable likelihood" of such survival.

At present, most obstetrician-gynecologists seem to consider viability of normal fetuses to occur somewhere in the range of twenty-two to twenty-four weeks. A question relevant to our discussion is whether there are any anomalies for which abortion beyond twenty-four weeks would justifiably be considered legal in all states because fetuses having those anomalies are legally nonviable. To explore this question, it will be helpful to consider several specific anomalies that might initially seem to justify a judgment of legal nonviability even after twenty-four weeks.

Let us consider, for example, anencephalic fetuses. Because anencephalics have an extremely poor prognosis for survival, I argued in an earlier article that they can reasonably be considered legally nonviable, even beyond twenty-four weeks.[21] However, recent cases have provided new evidence concerning our technological capability of keeping anencephalic infants legally alive. First, there were reports of several anencephalic infants being kept alive for a week or longer following birth by means of respirator support and other measures associated with intensive care.[22] More recently, two cases were reported in which anencephalic infants were kept alive for seven and ten months, respectively, without the use of prolonged respirator support.[23] In another case, an anencephalic infant was kept alive even longer by means of interventions including respirator support.[24] These reports call into question the previously held view that it is unlikely that an anencephalic infant can be kept alive for any extended period of time.

The possibility of respirator support for an anencephalic infant, together with the vagueness of the Supreme Court's definition of viability, creates a practical problem for the physician who would perform an abortion of an anencephalic fetus after twenty-four weeks. The problem is that it is not clear whether a court of law would consider this to be the abortion of a nonviable fetus. This creates a legal risk for the physician who would perform abortion in such circumstances. If such risks materialize, the well-being of the physician can be adversely affected and, as I pointed out above, the physician's well-being is one of the factors that the ethical framework considers relevant. In my view, the risks involved are serious enough that a prudent physician would be well advised not to perform abortions of anencephalic fetuses after twenty-four weeks, unless there is a separate justification in a particular case based on protecting maternal health or life. This implies that, on practical grounds, abortion of an anencephalic fetus should not be presented as a locally available option, unless there is a valid argument based on maternal health or life, or the jurisdiction in question permits postviability abortions for reasons other than maternal health and life.

We might also consider trisomy 13 and 18 syndromes, two of the most common types of genetic anomalies that are, with rare exception, incompatible with long-term survival.[25] Again, the vagueness of the legal definition of viability creates problems for the physician who would perform abortion after twenty-four weeks. In some cases, infants with these syndromes survive for months after birth. Thirty-one percent of infants with trisomy 13 syndrome survive six months or longer, and 18 percent survive beyond the first year. There is one reported case of an adult at age thirty-three. Fifty percent of infants with trisomy 18 syndrome survive two months or longer, and 10 percent survive beyond the first year.[26] Would a court of law consider survival for several months to constitute "sustained survival"? How likely would such survival have to be in order for a court to find that there is a "reasonable likelihood" of survival? Again, there is a legal risk to the physician, which might be quite significant.

In order for there to be relatively little legal risk to the physician, given the current legal framework, it seems that a case would have to contain several features. First, the anomaly would have to be one for which survival for more than a brief period after birth is impossible, even with technological interventions currently available. Second, the anomaly would have to be one that can be diagnosed with a relatively high degree of reliability, so that one could plausibly maintain that, having made the diagnosis, there is a "reasonable likelihood" that the infant could not be kept alive for a "sustained" period of time. Given current technological capabilities, there are few, if any, anomalies for which these features are present. This implies that, currently, abortion for serious fetal anomalies after twenty-four weeks would only rarely, if ever, be a legal option, except in the few states mentioned above that permit abortions after viability for reasons other than maternal health and life.[27]

Clinical Situations after Viability

After legal viability, the focus of decision making turns from abortion to the other three options—the aggressive, nonaggressive, and balancing approaches. In this section, I would like to explore the question of what recommendations the physician should make, if any, concerning these options when fetal anomalies are present after viability. Deciding which option to recommend involves, primarily, weighing maternal well-being against fetal well-being. A number of casuistic factors are relevant to the question of how priorities should be assigned to these two conflicting values. These include the following: the degree of reliability of the diagnosis of fetal malformation; the fetal prognosis concerning survival and cognitive development, if the diagnosis is correct and an aggressive approach is taken; the likelihood and magnitude of benefits to the fetus that would be expected to result from interventions carried out for the sake of the fetus; the likelihood and magnitude of potential harms to the pregnant woman that would be involved in such interventions; the likelihood and magnitude of potential harms to the fetus that would be involved in procedures carried out for the sake of the pregnant woman; and whether a procedure being contemplated for the sake of the pregnant woman would constitute killing the fetus. The variation in these factors from case to case depends largely on the type of fetal anomaly (or anomalies) in question, the pregnant woman's own medical condition, and the particular interventions being considered. The recommendations that are justifiable can vary with these factors, and perhaps the best way to illustrate this is to consider selected examples of fetal anomalies. My purpose in the following discussion is not to provide a comprehensive account of all commonly occurring anomalies but to illustrate how the ethical framework can usefully be applied to decisions in these sorts of cases. One test of the validity of the framework is its helpfulness in dealing with such cases.

HYDROCEPHALY

Hydrocephaly consists of an abnormal accumulation of cerebrospinal fluid within the ventricles of the brain. This condition accounts for approximately 12 percent of all serious malformations at birth.[28] The fluid can raise intracranial pressure, and if the pressure is persistently high it destroys cerebral white matter and causes permanent disabilities, including mental retardation, problems with motor function such as inability to walk, and blindness in some cases.[29] A large fluid volume can expand the cranium, making normal passage of the fetal head through the birth canal impossible. In 70 to 86 percent of cases, hydrocephaly is accompanied by other major anomalies; these include heart defects, brain malformations and, in about one-third of cases, myelomeningocele.[30] In one series, ten of twenty-four fetuses had defects incompatible with long-term survival detected in utero.[31]

Although placement of a ventriculoamniotic shunt in utero is possible, this approach has had limited success and currently is regarded as experimental. For these reasons, it is not considered to be the best approach for fetuses beyond approximately thirty-two weeks' gestational age. Delivery as soon as the lungs are mature, followed by shunt insertion, may be more favorable for these fetuses than the in utero shunting procedure.[32] In decisions about obstetric management, an important question concerns how to deliver the fetus in this later stage of gestation.

There are two main methods of delivery of the hydrocephalic fetus. One method attempts to minimize fetal injury. It involves delivery soon after the lungs are mature, so that the infant's condition can be better assessed and treatment can be started, including ventriculo-peritoneal shunt insertion if needed to drain the excess fluid. The timing of delivery would take into account the risks of prematurity, balanced against the risk of brain damage due to prolongation of the hydrocephalus. This approach utilizes cesarean section when the fetal head is larger than the pelvic opening, in order to avoid trauma to the fetus that would be caused by attempted vaginal delivery. An *aggressive* approach to management would involve this method of delivery. A drawback of this delivery method is exposure of the woman to the risks of surgical delivery. The maternal death rate due to cesarean section is .6 to 9 per 10,000 procedures, representing a two- to elevenfold increased risk compared to vaginal delivery.[33] Additional complications of cesarean section include infection, hemorrhage, and injuries to the urinary tract. Infrequently, there is uterine bleeding that can be controlled only by hysterectomy. In one report, significant complications other than death occurred in 21 percent of cesarean sections, compared to 4 percent of vaginal deliveries.[34] Others estimate that nonfatal complications occur in about 12 percent of cesarean sections overall.[35]

The alternative method attempts to minimize physical risks to the pregnant woman by avoiding cesarean section. This approach involves continuing the pregnancy until labor begins spontaneously, followed by vaginal delivery. If the fetal head is too large to pass through the pelvis, a needle can be inserted into the head and cerebrospinal fluid extracted in order to reduce the head size. However, this cephalocentesis almost always results in stillbirth or neonatal death within a few days, due to the rapid decompression of the head or needle-induced hemorrhage.[36] A review of cases involving cephalocentesis in which outcome was reported showed that for thirty-eight of forty-one fetuses, death followed within a short period.[37] Another report confirmed the injurious nature of the procedure by documenting massive hemorrhage in one case and heart rate changes in two cases indicative of fetal distress, including late decelerations, loss of beat-to-beat variability, low heart rate, and cardiac arrest.[38] It is conceivable that in the future a method of decompression will be developed that does not have such unfavorable consequences. At present, however, the risks to the fetus are severe. The *nonaggressive* approach to management would utilize this delivery method, and the *balancing* approach might use it, as well.

In comparing the two methods of delivery, it is helpful to consider the likely outcome for the fetus when atraumatic delivery and full treatment efforts are provided. The outcomes for fetuses with prenatally detected hydrocephalus have been described in several reports.[39] A total of 254 cases were reported in the studies cited, and 89 infants survived. However, not all the fetuses and neonates who died received aggressive management. To estimate the outcome after aggressive treatment, it is necessary to exclude the following types of cases from the reported data: abortion after detection of hydrocephalus early in gestation; delivery using cephalocentesis; prenatal detection of anomalies incompatible with survival; and cases reported in a manner suggesting nonaggressive management. Given these exclusions, the combined data show that 89 of 129 fetuses (69 percent) survived. Among the 76 survivors followed, 41 were handicapped (54 percent). It should be noted that these estimates are biased by the selection of fetuses who are treated. Generally, the prognosis is less favorable when additional anomalies are present. When the prognosis is known to be poor, vaginal delivery with cephalocentesis, if needed, is usually chosen. Thus, these estimates are based on a subgroup that probably tends to have less severe malformations compared to the entire group of fetuses reported.

Given the above considerations, the choice of delivery method has important consequences for the well-being of mother and fetus. Moreover, the risks to the mother are not confined to physical harms associated with delivery. There is a possibility, especially with cesarean section, of infant survival with permanent handicaps, depending on the presence of other anomalies and the severity of the damage caused by hydrocephalus. A number of studies have documented ways in which the well-being of parents can be adversely affected by the task of caring for a handicapped child.[40] On the other hand, a question that should be raised is whether cephalocentesis is ever ethically justifiable, given that the procedure is likely to constitute killing.

One of the casuistic factors is the degree of reliability of the diagnosis of fetal malformation. The importance of this factor can be seen by considering that it would not be justifiable to recommend the nonaggressive approach because of a suspected fetal malformation when the diagnosis is unreliable, particularly when the nonaggressive approach is likely to cause significant harm to the fetus. The diagnosis of hydrocephaly is made by ultrasound examination and involves comparing the width of the lateral ventricles with the hemispheric width of the fetal head. The diagnosis can be made with a relatively high degree of reliability.[41] With regard to other anomalies that might also be present, the reliability of diagnosis can vary, depending on the anomaly. This variability can affect the recommendation that should be made, as we shall see.

Another important casuistic factor is the fetal prognosis concerning survival and cognitive development if the diagnosis is correct and an aggressive approach is taken. Clinically, there is a spectrum of cases, with fetal prognosis varying from poor to relatively favorable and often characterized by uncertainty. To organize my discussion, I shall consider different categories of prognosis.

Let me begin with cases having the most favorable prognosis. Generally, fetuses for whom a thorough search reveals no other anomalies — fetuses with "isolated" hydrocephaly — tend to have a relatively favorable prognosis. However, sometimes even fetuses with isolated hydrocephaly have a poor outcome, particularly if there is elevated intracranial pressure of long-standing duration.[42] Thus, in the absence of specific evidence that the hydrocephaly is long-standing, a fetus with isolated hydrocephaly can be regarded as having a relatively favorable prognosis. Such a fetus would reasonably be considered to be sentient, viable, and having a potential for self-consciousness, given that we are discussing fetuses that are relatively advanced in gestation (approximately thirty-two weeks or later). Thus, it would have the same degree of similarity to the paradigm as a normal fetus of the same gestational age, and it would have a conferred moral standing that is very close to, but slightly less than, that of normative personhood. The principle of avoiding killing would have relatively strong weight with respect to the fetus in such a case. Because cephalocentesis would likely constitute killing, it should be avoided and cesarean section should be recommended. This conclusion is also supported by considerations of beneficence toward the fetus and pregnant woman. Because the fetus's conferred moral standing is relatively high, the physician's duty to the fetus to act beneficently toward it has considerable weight. Although the fetal prognosis is somewhat uncertain, the fetus has a chance for healthy survival. Even if mild or moderate handicaps later become evident, aggressive management is much better for the fetus than cephalocentesis. Moreover, the potential harm of cesarean section for the pregnant woman seems to be considerably less than the potential harm of cephalocentesis for the fetus. Thus, the overall risk of harm to mother and fetus would be minimized by the aggressive approach.

In this type of case, the pregnant woman often wants to do whatever is best for the fetus. If she agrees to cesarean delivery, then the physician should support her choice, but if she is reluctant to accept cesarean section, then the physician should encourage her to reconsider. Because part of the physician's role is to assist the patient in making a well-informed decision, the physician should try to help the patient who refuses cesarean delivery to understand the pros and cons. An adamant refusal of cesarean section by the mother would raise the issue of coerced treatment, a topic that will be addressed in Chapter 9.[43]

At the opposite extreme are cases in which the fetal prognosis is least favorable. The justification of cephalocentesis is strongest when additional anomalies have been detected with a high degree of reliability that are incompatible with long-term survival. An example would be thanatophoric dysplasia with cloverleaf skull.[44] In this type of situation, the physician should recommend nonaggressive management, including cephalocentesis if needed. A strong argument justifying this conclusion is needed, given the seriousness of killing, and such an argument is based on several considerations. First, the degree of harm to the fetus that might result from cephalocentesis is considerably diminished by the fact that the anomalies preclude long-term survival. Second, the pain and risks of cesarean section for the mother would be avoided. It might be objected that although such fetuses have a fatal condition, nevertheless it is wrong to kill them to prevent nonlethal harm to the mother. In reply, the similarity with the paradigm is diminished because such fetuses lack the potential to become self-conscious. They lack this potential because they will not survive to a stage of development at which self-consciousness could be said to exist. Because the similarity is diminished, these fetuses have a moral standing that is diminished compared to normative personhood, and the principle of avoiding killing also has diminished strength. This does not mean that killing should be taken lightly in such cases. However, these considerations support the view that the rule against killing has sufficiently attenuated force in such circumstances to justify killing the fetus to prevent significant but nonlethal harm to the mother.

Cephalocentesis also is justifiable when anomalies have been detected with a high degree of reliability having a prognosis that can vary between death and, at best, survival with profound cognitive deficit. Examples include trisomy 13 and 18 syndromes and alobar holoprosencephaly.[45] In this type of case, also, the physician should recommend the nonaggressive approach. The ethical justification of this recommendation is based on the fact that it is highly unlikely that cesarean section would significantly benefit the fetus, and surgical risks for the woman would be avoided. Also, in such cases survival would be accompanied by cognitive impairments so severe that self-consciousness would never occur. Thus, the fetuses in question have a diminished similarity to the paradigm. Because of the diminished moral status, the principle of avoiding killing has reduced force in such cases, again justifying killing to prevent significant nonlethal harm to the woman.

Between the extremes of good-prognosis and poor-prognosis cases, there is a spectrum of varying fetal prognosis. Close to the poor-prognosis cases, there are cases involving serious malformations in which there is more uncertainty concerning whether either death or profound cognitive deficit will occur. This state of affairs might arise because the long-term outcome cannot be reliably predicted, as in some cases involving Dandy-Walker syndrome, for example, or the diagnosis is less than highly reliable, as in renal agenesis.[46] Decisions in these borderline cases are perhaps the most difficult, and it is reasonable to consider additional casuistic factors in deciding whether a recommendation of cephalocentesis is justifiable. These include the likelihood and magnitude of potential harms to the pregnant woman that would be involved in cesarean delivery. In particular, the presence of conditions that increase the operative risks for the woman would strengthen the argument for vaginal delivery. If she is obese, for example, it is likely that the operative wound would take longer to heal and there would be an increased risk of wound infection.[47] If she has chorioamnionitis (infection of membranes surrounding the fetus), then it would be desirable to avoid cesarean delivery in order to prevent further spread of the infection.[48] If she has an impairment in the mechanism of blood coagulation, then it would be preferable, other things being equal, to avoid surgical delivery.[49] Even when additional casuistic factors are considered, however, there will be cases in which there is no clear answer. In these gray-area cases, I suggest that the physician should lean toward the avoidance of killing.

Finally, there are situations in which the prognosis is better than that of the borderline but worse than that of the best-prognosis cases. These are instances in which additional anomalies are present, but not ones that are likely to result in death or severe cognitive deficit. An example is the case described at the beginning of this chapter, involving head enlargement and spina bifida. In such cases, the physician should recommend the aggressive approach because the potential harm of cephalocentesis to the fetus is considerable. Admittedly, the potential harms for the mother arising from cesarean delivery, particularly any long-term harms associated with raising a handicapped child, might be greater in these instances than in the best-prognosis cases because there is a greater likelihood of survival of a handicapped child. However, the fetuses in question would have the same moral status as normal fetuses with the same gestational age. Thus, the principle of avoiding killing has considerable force in such cases and strongly supports an aggressive approach.

OCCIPITAL ENCEPHALOCELE

An encephalocele is a herniation of the brain and meninges through a defect in the skull, resulting in a sac-like structure. When the defect contains only meninges, it is referred to as a cranial meningocele. Encephaloceles can be diagnosed in utero by ultrasound, but not with complete reliability in all cases. In two studies, a false-positive result was found in one of nine cases and in one of five cases, respectively.[50] The outcomes for fetuses with prenatally detected encephalocele have been described in a number of reports.[51] Excluding those involving abortion, a total of 251 cases were reported in the studies cited, and 131 of the infants survived (52 percent). Among 129 survivors for whom developmental outcomes were reported, 91 had handicaps of varying degrees (71 percent). Factors affecting the outcome include the size of the herniation, the occurrence of microcephaly, and the presence of other anomalies, including hydrocephaly.[52] In those with a large brain herniation (approximately one-half the diameter of the fetal head or larger) and microcephaly, the fetus usually dies. In the occasional instance of long-term survival, there usually is minimal cognitive development.[53] In those with small herniations (up to several centimeters in diameter) and normal head size, the prognosis is more variable, ranging from normal mental and physical development to moderate handicaps.[54]

The recommendation that the physician should make depends on the casuistic factors, including the severity of the anomaly. Let us first consider the cases in which the prognosis is most favorable, those involving small herniations and no other detected anomalies. The fetuses in these cases are likely to survive, and they have the potential to become self-conscious. They seem to have the same degree of similarity to the paradigm as normal fetuses of the same gestational age. During the stage of gestation now under consideration, the postviability period, these fetuses are relatively advanced in development and should be regarded as having a conferred moral status that is very close to, although slightly less than, that of normative personhood. In such cases, the physician should recommend the aggressive approach. This would include, for example, cesarean section if fetal distress occurs.[55] This conclusion is supported by several considerations. First, because of the favorable prognosis, the fetus has a significant potential to benefit from therapeutic interventions. Second, because of the fetus's conferred moral status, the physician has a relatively strong duty to the fetus to act beneficently toward it. Third, although aggressive management might pose risks to the health of the pregnant woman, those risks generally are small compared to the risks to the fetus associated with the nonaggressive approach. Thus, the risks to the woman are ones that it is reasonable to recommend that she take, given the significant potential benefits for the fetus.

When the prognosis is favorable, as in the cases being considered, the woman typically will want to do everything possible to promote the well-being of the fetus. If she agrees to take an aggressive approach, the physician should support her choice. If she prefers a nonaggressive approach, the physician should encourage her to reconsider.

At the other extreme are the worst-prognosis cases, involving large herniations and microcephaly. Because of their exceedingly poor prognosis, these fetuses lack the potential to become self-conscious. Because of their diminished similarity with the paradigm, they have a diminished moral standing compared to normal fetuses near term. The physician should recommend the nonaggressive approach to obstetric management, including avoidance of cesarean section, in such cases. This approach is ethically justifiable, based on several considerations. First, the likelihood and magnitude of potential benefits to the fetus from aggressive interventions are relatively small, due to the poor fetal prognosis. Second, the physician's duty to the fetus to act beneficently toward the fetus has reduced strength because of the fetus's diminished moral status. Third, risks to the health of the pregnant woman would be avoided.

Sometimes the pregnant woman will request an aggressive approach even though the fetal prognosis is very poor. Such requests might be based on a desire to deliver a live infant even though the woman realizes that there would not be prolonged survival after birth. It is conceivable that such a request might be made in a case involving severe encephalocele. In this type of case, it would be appropriate for the physician to attempt to persuade the woman to change her mind. If she is adamant, then the physician should attempt to persuade her to agree to a balancing approach. This might involve, for example, repositioning and oxygen therapy in the event of fetal distress, but withholding cesarean section.[56] This would constitute taking steps to bring about live birth but stopping short of those measures posing relatively greater risks to the woman. Such a negotiated agreement would result in the physician having certain limited obligations *to the woman* to act beneficently toward the fetus.

Other cases are between the extremes of most-favorable and very poor prognoses. Fetuses in these cases have a chance for survival, although individual cases will be characterized by considerable uncertainty concerning the prognosis for survival and cognitive development. It seems reasonable to regard these fetuses as retaining the capacity for sentience. Some might have the potential to become self-conscious, although during pregnancy it cannot be predicted reliably which ones would have such potential. In these cases, it is less clear what recommendations should be made. It would be reasonable to consider additional casuistic factors, including the likelihood and magnitude of potential harms to the pregnant woman that would be involved in aggressive interventions. For example, if conditions are present in a given case that increase the operative risks for the woman, this might tip the balance in favor of recommending vaginal rather than cesarean delivery in the event of fetal distress. Even when additional casuistic factors are considered, there will be cases in which neither the aggressive nor the nonaggressive approach is clearly preferable. In such situations, it seems reasonable for the physician to present in a nondirective manner the aggressive, nonaggressive, and balancing approaches for the pregnant woman to consider. If asked for a recommendation, it would seem reasonable for the physician to suggest the middle-ground balancing approach. In some cases, this approach might involve, for example, exposing the woman to risks of tocolysis but avoiding the somewhat greater risks associated with cesarean delivery.

ANENCEPHALY

Anencephalic fetuses lack a functioning cerebral cortex. As such, they do not have the anatomical structures necessary for self-consciousness. Moreover, the prognosis for survival is poor. Most of them are stillborn, and among those born alive, death usually occurs within twenty-four hours if there are no aggressive interventions such as respirator support. In the absence of such interventions, death almost always occurs within two weeks.[57] Methods used to diagnose anencephaly in utero include ultrasonography and measurement of elevated levels of alpha-fetoprotein and acetylcholinesterase in the amniotic fluid. The condition can be diagnosed in utero with a very high degree of reliability.[58]

Because anencephalic fetuses irreversibly lack consciousness, they are unable to experience pain or other sensations. This lack of sentience, together with the lack of potential for self-consciousness, means that they have a diminished similarity with the paradigm. This implies that they have a diminished moral standing, compared to normative personhood. When a fetus has anencephaly, the physician should recommend the nonaggressive approach to obstetric management. The ethical justification of this recommendation is based on several considerations. First, because these fetuses lack sentience, as well as the potential for sentience, they lack the capacity to be harmed or benefited in any way; aggressive interventions cannot possibly benefit them. Second, in the absence of maternal indications for intervening, any aggressive interventions would create unnecessary risks for the pregnant woman, and such risks should be avoided.

In this chapter, the view that fetal moral standing is related to the degree of similarity to the paradigm of descriptive persons has entered into the discussion in several ways. First, it helps explain why abortion before viability is ethically justifiable. Although the justification of previable abortion is based on considerations of maternal autonomy, maternal well-being, and fetal moral standing, the precise reason why previable fetuses lack personhood status is a matter of controversy. According to the view presented here, viability is not a criterion of personhood. Rather, what is relevant is that the previable fetus lacks a number of important similarities to the paradigm. Second, the view in question helps explain why cephalocentesis, which often would constitute killing the postviable fetus, is sometimes ethically justifiable. Killing requires a strong justification, and I have argued that when the fetus lacks the conferred moral standing of normative personhood, the principle of avoiding killing lacks full force. This together with other casuistic factors can justify cephalocentesis in certain cases. Third, when anomalies diminish a fetus's similarity to the paradigm, the physician's obligation to the fetus to act beneficently toward it is diminished in strength as well. This can play a role in the ethical justification of a recommendation for nonaggressive management in some cases.

The problem of deciding what recommendations a physician should make illustrates the usefulness of a casuistic approach to decision making in the clinical setting. I have tried to identify morally relevant casuistic factors that can vary from case to case. The process of reasoning that I have outlined in this chapter can be applied to other types of fetal anomalies not explicity discussed here. The conclusions reached for other anomalies would depend on the degree to which these casuistic factors are present in a given case.

9

Coercive Interventions during Pregnancy

Two cases dramatically illustrate the issue of coercive interventions for the sake of the fetus. In the first case, reported in 1981 by Watson A. Bowes, Jr., and Brad Selgestad, a thirty-three-year-old woman was admitted to the hospital in labor with a term fetus.[1] During labor, the fetal heart rate monitor showed late decelerations and loss of beat-to-beat variability, evidence that the fetus was not getting sufficient oxygen. The amniotic fluid was initially clear but later became meconium-stained, providing confirmation of fetal hypoxia. Repositioning the woman and giving her oxygen did not improve the monitor tracing.[2] She was told that an emergency cesarean section should be performed to prevent brain damage or death to the fetus. The woman, who had undergone surgery earlier in pregnancy for gall bladder disease, refused to have a cesarean section, stating that she was afraid of the surgery. The patient's mother and sister and the father of the fetus were present, and all of them attempted to persuade the patient to change her mind, but were unsuccessful. At that point, the physician was considering seeking a court order authorizing cesarean delivery without the woman's consent.

The second case occurred at my institution and involved an eighteen-year-year old woman at twenty-five weeks' gestation with a chronic placental abruption that had resulted in two bleeding episodes. Also, her amniotic membranes had ruptured prematurely, and she was a cocaine user. She was admitted to the hospital, transfused with three units of packed red blood cells, and treated with steroids in an attempt to promote fetal lung maturity in the event that there would be an early delivery. Continued hospitalization was considered necessary in order to monitor several problems. First, the placental abruption could result in another bleeding episode. Heavy bleeding could cause serious problems for mother and fetus, including maternal shock or coagulation defects and fetal exsanguination. Second, ruptured membranes significantly increase the risk of fetal infection, and hospitalization would permit close monitoring for signs of infection, which could be followed by treatment.[3] These reasons for remaining in the hospital were explained to the patient, but after several days she left the hospital against medical advice. The physicians suspected that she left in order to obtain cocaine. The physicians, who were greatly concerned about the patient's behavior, debated whether they should seek a court order for involuntary hospitalization.[4]

In the case described by Bowes and Selgestad, a court order was requested and a judge presided at a hearing held in the patient's hospital room. These proceedings resulted in a court order authorizing cesarean delivery. Upon issuance of the order, the woman reluctantly became more cooperative. Without resistance from her, a cesarean section was performed six and a half hours after she had initially refused it. Upon delivery, the infant had only moderate signs of distress, recovered promptly, and at eight months follow-up was growing and developing normally. This was one of the first times that a court had ordered a cesarean section of a mentally competent woman for the sake of the fetus. It led to court-ordered interventions by other physicians and a flood of commentary on the ethics and legality of such actions.

Coerced cesareans have now been performed for a variety of medical reasons, including fetal distress, previous cesarean section, placenta previa, failed progress of labor, and placental abruption.[5] Courts also have ordered maternal blood transfusions for life-threatening hemorrhage, fetal transfusions for Rh sensitization, and hospital detention for control of diabetes.[6] Moreover, legal actions have been taken against women who use cocaine or other drugs during pregnancy, including at least fifty attempts at prosecution.[7] In a highly publicized Florida case in 1989, Jennifer Johnson was prosecuted after two successive children born fourteen months apart tested positive for cocaine at birth. She was convicted of child abuse and delivery of drugs to a minor, based on the supposed transplacental passage of a cocaine derivative immediately after birth. Her sentence included mandatory drug treatment and a requirement that, if she became pregnant again, she must notify her probation officer and comply with a court-approved prenatal care program.[8]

Coerced intervention for the sake of the fetus has become a dominant issue in obstetric ethics and certainly one of the most controversial. This chapter addresses the question of whether coercive interventions imposed on mentally competent pregnant women are ever ethically and legally justifiable, and, if so, in what types of situations.

Applying the Ethical Framework

Several ethical values are especially relevant to this issue, including the autonomy and well-being of the pregnant woman and the well-being of the fetus and the child it might become. The pregnant woman and physician have obligations to promote the well-being of the fetus, and the physician also has obligations to respect and promote the autonomy and well-being of the woman. The autonomy and well-being of the physician are also pertinent, particularly because actions might be contemplated that threaten the ethical integrity of the physician or involve risks of legal liability. Although many commentators focus on the above-mentioned values, additional values can be relevant, including the well-being of other family members and the well-being of pregnant women as a group.

In most cases in which coercive interventions are being considered, the fetus is relatively advanced in gestation. Such fetuses have a moral status that is close to, but slightly less strong than, normative personhood. Moreover, it is not only for the fetus's sake that coercive interventions are considered; the well-being of the child the fetus will become, assuming it survives, is also at stake. It is usually presumed that at some point the surviving child will acquire normative personhood status, so we are concerned about the interests of a possible future person. These two factors taken together—the relatively high moral status of the fetus itself and the full moral status of a *possible* future person—support the view that serious weight should be given to fetal interests.

Similar comments can be made concerning the pregnant woman's *obligation* to promote the interests of her fetus. As noted in Chapter 3, the fetus's moral standing has an effect on this obligation. As fetal moral standing increases, this parental obligation becomes stronger. For a fetus that is relatively advanced in gestation, this obligation is relatively strong. Moreover, if there is going to be a future child with normative personhood status, the woman has a parental obligation to avoid actions that would be harmful to the child. These considerations support the claim that the woman's obligation is serious.

It is tempting to think that because the woman has a serious obligation to promote the welfare of the fetus, it is ethically justifiable to force her to fulfill that obligation. However, this conclusion does not automatically follow.

Depending on the obligations and circumstances in question, forcing people to fulfill their obligations might have negative consequences that overshadow the benefits of such coercion. Therefore, before drawing a conclusion, it would be necessary to consider the pros and cons of enforcing a given obligation. Rather than providing a solution, recognition that the pregnant woman has obligations to the fetus allows us to formulate the issue in another way: what we are exploring is whether it is ever ethically and legally justifiable to force the pregnant woman to fulfill her obligations to the fetus.

The modified casuistic approach provides a framework for resolving value conflicts. It holds that for some issues the prioritization of values should take place in the context of specific cases, and for other issues the prioritization is considered to hold for all cases. As indicated in Chapter 4, this approach leaves open the possibility that, for some issues, prioritizing should take place in the context of specific cases, but with a strong presumption in favor of certain ethical values. I shall argue that such a presumption arises with respect to the issue of coerced interventions during pregnancy.

Presumption Favoring Maternal Autonomy

In the extensive literature on forced maternal treatment, a number of arguments have been put forward against such interventions. These arguments raise such serious concerns that, taken together, they support the view that there is a strong presumption in favor of the pregnant woman's autonomy over the fetus's well-being. To put it differently, there is a strong presumption against forcing the pregnant woman to fulfill her obligations to the fetus. Let us consider these arguments.

The first argument applies specifically to interventions that would violate the bodily integrity of the pregnant woman. The bodily integrity of mentally competent individuals who are persons in the descriptive sense is an extremely important ethical value. Control over one's body is a crucial aspect of self-determination. Only the most compelling of reasons would justify a significant violation of the physical integrity of a person's body. Moreover, allowing women to have control over their bodies is particularly crucial, given the importance of the self-determination of women in gaining social, political, and economic equality, as discussed in Chapter 2.

Second, these cases *typically* do not involve *actual* third parties with normative personhood status who are put in harm's way by the pregnant woman's actions. The fetus does not have full normative personhood status, and the potential child who *would* have normative personhood status does not yet exist and might never come into being. Thus, prevention of harm to the fetus or potential child, although a serious concern, does not have quite the degree of moral weight that prevention of harm to an actual individual with normative personhood status would have.

Third, in the absence of a strong presumption against forced interventions, the burden of coerced treatment is likely to fall disproportionately upon minority women. Evidence for this is provided in a report by Veronika E. B. Kolder and colleagues.[9] In seventeen (81 percent) of twenty-one reported cases in which court orders were sought for forced treatment, the patients were black, Asian, or Hispanic. The reasons for this discriminatory practice have not been well documented but probably have to do with cultural differences and language barriers between physicians and minority patients. A presumption against coerced interventions would help reduce this discriminatory burden by reducing the absolute number of interventions and by requiring obstetricians to give more serious attention to the reasons why minority women refuse proposed treatments. It is better to develop innovative strategies for identifying women's reasons and attempting to persuade them than to force treatment.

Fourth, when forced treatment occurs, it can disrupt the relationship between the specific patient and physician. If the patient becomes alienated from the physician, she might be less inclined to cooperate with further efforts to provide care to her. It would be desirable to minimize the number of such occurrences.

Fifth, unless there is a widely recognized strong presumption against invasions of maternal liberty, it is likely that coercive interventions would be sufficiently common to be perceived as quite threatening by women seeking health care. There is evidence for this in the fact that such interventions were more common before a strong legal presumption against them was set forth in the case of *In re A. C.*[10] The report by Kolder and coworkers identified twenty-one cases in which court orders were sought for forced treatment in the United Stated during the five-year period prior to 1986.[11] After the *In re A. C.* case in 1990, court-ordered interventions decreased in frequency; I am aware of only one publicized attempt to perform a court-ordered cesarean section during this period, and the court declined to issue a court order in that case.[12] Evidence that coerced interventions have been perceived as threatening to women, particularly during the period before *In re A. C.*, can be found in the large number of articles written by women identifying the threatening aspects of these practices.[13] When women feel threatened in this way, there could be negative consequences: the relationship of trust between obstetricians generally and their patients could be undermined to some extent, and some women could be less inclined to seek the care of obstetricians or comply with their recommendations. This could have harmful effects on the health of women and their fetuses. Admittedly, there is uncertainty concerning the extent to which these adverse consequences would occur. Thus, this argument might not be as forceful as the preceding ones, but to the extent that it raises a legitimate concern, it gives support to those arguments. All five arguments taken together provide grounds for the view that there should be a strong presumption against invasions of maternal liberty.

In addition to this presumption, a number of casuistic factors are relevant to the question of whether a coerced intervention would be justifiable in a given case. Specifically, the argument against intervening becomes stronger as the risk to the life or health of the woman posed by the intervention increases, as the degree of invasion of the woman's bodily integrity increases, and as the extent to which the intervention infringes the woman's liberty increases. On the other hand, the argument supporting intervention becomes stronger as the degree of harm to the fetus that would be prevented by the intervention in- creases, and as the likelihood that the intervention would prevent harm to the fetus increases. This is not meant to be an exhaustive list of the casuistic factors, but only some of the main ones. Because these factors can vary from case to case, the argument for coerced intervention can vary in strength.

The presumption in favor of maternal autonomy should not be taken to mean that intervention is never justifiable. Cases can arise, although they are seemingly rare, in which the considerations supporting intervention are com- pelling. To see this, let us consider a scenario in which court-ordered treatment appears to be ethically justifiable. As a first step toward identifying this sce- nario, let us consider the case of *Application of Jamaica Hospital,* which occurred in 1985 in New York City. This case involved a patient at eighteen weeks' gestational age with esophageal varices resulting in internal bleeding.[14] The bleeding became life-threatening and the physician recommended blood transfusions. However, the patient refused transfusions because of her re- ligious beliefs as a Jehovah's Witness. The patient was single and was the mother of ten children. The only next of kin was a sister who was unavailable. The physician and hospital sought a court order authorizing blood transfu- sions for the woman. A hearing was held and the physician testified that transfusions were necessary to save the life of the mother and the fetus. The judge granted a court order and stated that the decision was based largely on the state's interest in protecting the life of the fetus.

The case I would like to consider is a variation of the *Jamaica Hospital* case. Let us suppose that a discussion with the patient reveals that there is no living father of the children and there is no one in her family who would be able to raise her children if she died.[15] Let us also suppose that the case involves a fetus near term, rather than at eighteen weeks' gestation. An ethical justification of court-ordered blood transfusions in this modified case can be given, based on several considerations. First, in choosing death, the patient would be abandoning her children, to use the law's terminology. They would experience the psychological trauma arising from death of a parent and would suffer the further harms associated with having no parent to care for them. Harm to others, in particular the children, is a casuistic factor that is highly relevant in this particular case. Second, the well-being of the fetus near term and of the possible child it might become deserves consideration. The magnitude and probability of harm to the fetus are relevant casuistic factors, and both are high in this case. Third, the degree of harm that would occur to the woman without the intervention is a casuistic factor that supports intervening in this case because there is a high probability of death without the transfusions. Fourth, if the woman dies, the community will have an increased burden associated with care of the ten children. Perhaps none of these factors alone would justify court-ordered transfusions in this case. However, all four considered together constitute a compelling argument for intervention. This case, in which the well-being of the children is an important consideration, illustrates the fact that sometimes more is at stake in maternal-fetal conflicts than the interests of the pregnant woman and fetus.

The Legal Framework

Before discussing further the conditions that must be satisfied in order for coerced intervention to be justifiable, it will be helpful to consider the current legal framework in the United States. In particular, two main features of the law are worth noting. First, the strong presumption in favor of maternal autonomy for which I argued is recognized in the law, having been set forth in the *In re A. C.* decision. Prior to this decision, court orders had authorized interventions in a number of cases, but in other cases judges had declined to issue such orders.[16] Moreover, before the case of A. C., only two potentially precedent-setting court of appeals decisions had been issued, *Jefferson v. Griffin Spalding County Hospital Authority* and *Raleigh Fitkin–Paul Morgan Memorial Hospital v. Anderson*.[17] It has been pointed out that *Raleigh Fitkin* should be regarded as having little value as a precedent because the opinion was extremely brief, with little policy discussion,[18] and the case was decided over three decades ago, when patients' legal rights to self-determination and bodily integrity were less prominent than they are today.[19] For similar reasons, *Jefferson* also should be regarded as having little weight as a precedent.[20] Thus, the cases before *In re A. C.* produced neither a consistent pattern of decision making by judges nor clear precedents.

The Court of Appeals decision in the case of A. C. was the first involving coerced maternal treatment in which a careful and thorough deliberative process was carried out; in almost all previous cases, the urgency of the clinical situation had called for a legal decision within a relatively short time. This urgency, in fact, precluded the possibility of involving the courts in some cases.[21] In *In re A. C.,* the medical decisions had been made, and the Court of Appeals was free to take a number of months to research the law and reach its decision, which helped make the case an important one.

In this case, Angela Carder was a twenty-eight-year-old married patient at twenty-six weeks' gestation. She was diagnosed as having a cancerous tumor that nearly filled her right lung. Her condition quickly deteriorated, and her doctors at George Washington University Hospital informed her that it was terminal. She agreed to palliative treatment in the hope of extending her life to at least twenty-eight weeks' gestation, based in part on the fact that her obstetricians preferred not to attempt delivery prior to twenty-eight weeks if possible. She was asked whether she still wanted the baby, and she said something to the effect of "I don't know. I think so." Her condition worsened and she was intubated. She was given sedatives to produce compliance with the ventilator. At that point, Ms. Carder was expected to live only a couple of days, and the fetus's condition was deteriorating. The hospital administrators decided to seek legal advice on whether to proceed with delivery. This led to a court hearing held at the hospital while the patient was sedated. Before sedation, she had agreed to cesarean delivery if needed at twenty-eight weeks, but there had been no discussion concerning delivery at the current twenty-six weeks. Before the hearing ended, the sedative wore off somewhat, and the obstetricians discussed cesarean delivery with her. She agreed to the procedure, but after a short period the obstetricians visited her again to confirm her consent, and this time she indicated that she did not want the cesarean. There was controversy over whether this was an informed, competent refusal, and the judge concluded that it still was not clear what the patient wanted. The family and obstetricians were opposed to the operation, but the judge issued an order authorizing it in an attempt to save the fetus. Cesarean delivery was performed, but the child lived only a few hours, and Ms. Carder died two days later.[22]

Because of the need for legal guidance for future cases, a full panel of judges of the Court of Appeals agreed to review the case. The appeals court held that the lower court had erred in ordering a cesarean section. The Court of Appeals outlined an approach to be followed by courts in such cases. According to this approach, a determination must be made concerning the mental competency of the patient. The court asserted that if she is competent, then "*in virtually all cases* the question of what is to be done is to be decided by the patient — the pregnant woman—on behalf of herself and the fetus."[23] If she is mentally incompetent, then her wishes must be inferred by the procedure of substituted judgment. The court stated that if her wishes are inferred in this manner, then "in virtually all cases the decision of the patient, albeit discerned through the mechanism of substituted judgment, will control. We do not quite foreclose the possibility that a conflicting state interest might be so compelling that the patient's wishes must yield, but we anticipate that such cases will be extremely rare and truly exceptional."[24] The lower court decision was overturned because the judge had failed to state explicitly whether the patient was incompetent and whether the legal doctrine of substituted judgment was being used. Thus, as pointed out by other commentators,[25] *In re A. C.* established a legal precedent that the mentally competent pregnant woman's decision concerning treatment almost always should prevail.[26]

The second main feature of the current legal framework concerns the level of risk that the woman legally can be forced to undergo. The case most pertinent to this question is *Thornburgh v. American College of Obstetricians and Gynecologists.*[27] This case was decided by the United States Supreme Court in 1986, and it involved the constitutionality of Pennsylvania's abortion law. The relevance of *Thornburgh* to the issue of forced maternal treatment has been pointed out by a number of lawyer-ethicists.[28] In *Roe v. Wade,* the Supreme Court had ruled that abortions must be allowed, even after viability, whenever they are necessary to preserve the life or health of the pregnant woman.[29] The Pennsylvania law in question stated that a physician performing such an abortion after viability must use the abortion technique that would provide the best opportunity for the unborn child to be aborted alive unless it would present a significantly greater medical risk to the pregnant woman's life or health.[30] The Supreme Court ruled that this part of the law was unconstitutional because in some cases it would require the pregnant woman to undergo increased risks. Specifically, the Court stated that it is unconstitutional to require the woman to undergo any increased risk for the sake of the fetus because doing so constitutes a barrier to her right to have an abortion.[31]

As legal commentators have pointed out, if it is unconstitutional to require the woman to assume increased risks for the sake of the fetus in the context of therapeutic abortion, then it would also seem to be unconstitutional to require her to undergo increased risks for the sake of the fetus in the context of nonabortion therapy.[32]

Let us consider an objection that might be raised against this conclusion. It might be claimed that because abortion is a constitutionally protected right, the abortion context is different legally from the context of treatment refusal. Thus, the argument goes, the suggested analogy does not hold, and statements made by the Court in the abortion context are not applicable to the context of therapy for fetal indications. In reply, the context of refusal of therapy for fetal indications also involves a constitutionally protected right — the right to refuse treatment. In *Cruzan v. Director, Missouri Department of Health*, the Supreme Court stated that there is a constitutionally protected liberty interest in refusing unwanted medical treatment.[33] In fact, language used by the Supreme Court and appellate courts suggests that the right to refuse medical treatment and the right to abortion are two aspects of a more fundamental right to self-determination — a right to self-rule concerning important decisions affecting one's life.[34]

To maintain that the Supreme Court statements in the abortion context do not carry over to the context of treatment refusal, one would have to claim that the legal right to refuse treatment is less weighty than the legal right to have an abortion. In other words, one would have to claim that fetal interests override the legal right to refuse treatment but do not override the right to abortion. However, it is not clear how one could satisfactorily defend that claim. Both rights are very important and are constitutionally protected. There does not seem to be any basis for claiming that one is more important than the other. Therefore, the argument that it is unconstitutional to require therapy for the sake of the fetus if it involves increased risks for the woman appears sound.[35]

Conditions for Justifiable Coerced Intervention

The strong ethical presumption against interference with maternal liberty, together with the legal precedent set in *In re A. C.*, support the view that coerced intervention would be justifiable both ethically and legally only in rare, exceptional circumstances. Moreover, any coerced interference that exposes the woman, on balance, to increased risks would be incompatible with the legal framework. For these reasons, the following view is defensible: Coercive interventions carried out upon a mentally competent pregnant woman would be ethically and legally justifiable provided two main conditions are met: (1) the intervention poses insignificant or no health risks to the woman or would promote her interest in life or health; and (2) there are reasons supporting intervention that are sufficiently compelling to override a strong presumption in favor of maternal autonomy.

The compelling reasons might vary, depending on the case, and would likely consist of multiple considerations. Examples of considerations include, but are not necessarily limited to: protecting fetal life; preventing serious harm to the fetus; preventing the abandonment of dependent children; protecting the mother's life; preventing harm to the mother's health; preserving the ethical integrity of the physician; and promoting the well-being of the community. Although some of these considerations alone might never justify coerced treatment, several together could do so in exceptional situations.

To further clarify this view, several points should be made. First, the autonomy and bodily integrity of obstetric patients almost always should be respected even if doing so means that harm is likely to occur to the fetus. Second, in addition to bodily integrity, maternal liberty is an important concern. Even though an intervention does not invade bodily integrity, if it is highly invasive of liberty, then it would be very difficult to justify. Third, use of physical force by physicians and other health professionals upon resistant, mentally competent pregnant women should be avoided. Such action is contrary to the role of health professionals, might increase the risks to the woman, and would undermine the relationship of trust between patients and physicians. Only lesser forms of coercion, such as bringing the moral and legal weight of a court order to bear upon her decision, would ever be justifiable. Fourth, advance discussions with the woman, when possible and appropriate, should be carried out in an attempt to identify and resolve value conflicts before they manifest themselves in crisis situations.[36] Fifth, the argument for intervention is strengthened if the patient's capacity to make an autonomous decision is significantly diminished.[37]

An important question is whether court-ordered cesarean section is ever ethically and legally justifiable. Some have argued that cesarean section is too invasive to be justifiable.[38] However, sometimes a cesarean is likely to promote significantly the woman's well-being. An example would involve placenta previa, for which cesarean section would significantly reduce the risk of maternal death. Thus, the invasiveness of the procedure can sometimes be offset by the expected benefits, suggesting that we should not try to draw a sharp line at a given level of invasiveness. Others have suggested that certain situations involving cesarean delivery are among the clearest examples of justifiable coerced maternal treatment. In particular, a number of clinicians have maintained that coerced cesarean section for complete placenta previa is justifiable.[39] However, there are difficulties with this view. Consider the case of Barbara Jeffries, a thirty-three-year-old Michigan woman who was diagnosed as having placenta previa. When she refused cesarean section on religious grounds, the doctor sought a court order. The judge issued orders for the police to transport Ms. Jeffries to the hospital and have her admitted. However, the police were unable to find her. Later it was learned that she had heard about the court order, and she and her family had fled the state.[40] As this case illustrates, seeking a court order might drive the patient away from the hospital. Another concern is that the patient might even try to have an out-of-hospital delivery.[41] These considerations undermine the view that a court order is *always* a sound approach to treatment refusal in cases of complete placenta previa, but they do not rule out the possibility that a forced cesarean might be justifiable in some cases of this type. It is conceivable, for example, that a given patient with complete placenta previa might be known to be unwilling or unable to flee or otherwise avoid medical care. These considerations support the view that coerced cesarean delivery is justifiable only in rare situations.[42]

Substance Abuse during Pregnancy

The case of Jennifer Johnson, discussed above, illustrates the coercion of pregnant women by the judicial system in an attempt to prevent substance abuse that would be harmful to the fetus. Studies indicate that from 7 to 31 percent of women in various obstetric populations in the United States are substance abusers, and these figures likely are conservative due to under-reporting.[43] Cocaine use can cause spontaneous abortion, in utero strokes, and placental abruption.[44] It also is associated with preterm labor and delivery, intrauterine growth retardation, congenital anomalies including cardiac, urinary, and neural tube defects, and increased infant mortality.[45] Cocaine-exposed infants often have withdrawal symptoms including irritability, restlessness, inability to sleep, incessant shrill crying, and, in severe cases, convulsions.[46] Long-term effects are believed to include learning disabilities.[47]

Despite these harms to fetuses, all of the arguments supporting a strong presumption against coercive medical interventions during pregnancy apply in the context of drug abuse, and additional arguments specific to the drug abuse context support this presumption. Consider, for example, the view that pregnant addicts should be held in state custody in detoxification centers.[48] One problem with this approach is that health care providers would be involved in reporting patients to authorities. If routinely followed, this approach would likely drive drug-using women away from prenatal care.[49] The approach also would highly invade the liberty of women, but because injury to the fetus might already have occurred, the degree of fetal benefit that would be obtained by detaining the woman would be unclear. Another problem in the United States is the shortage of facilities to provide such treatment. Many drug rehabilitation programs refuse to accept pregnant women due to fear of liability for injured babies.[50] Moreover, coerced treatment for drug addiction sometimes does not receive the cooperation of the patient.[51] These considerations support the view that detention is not a favorable approach.[52]

The arguments against coercive interventions can be illustrated using the case discussed at the beginning of this chapter, involving the patient with chronic placental abruption who used cocaine. Seeking a court order for detention would unavoidably involve bringing the patient's cocaine use to the attention of the authorities and would likely alienate the patient from her health care providers. Also, hospital detention is highly invasive of liberty, and the probability that harm to the fetus would be prevented does not seem to be great enough to justify such drastic measures in this case. Moreover, even if the patient is detained, there would be no guarantee that the fetus would be free of serious medical problems caused by the cocaine use that had already occurred. A preferable approach would involve persuasion and efforts to maintain a good physician-patient relationship. The woman should be counseled concerning the risks to the fetus and herself and strongly urged to return promptly to the hospital. Threats and confrontation are best avoided, to prevent undermining the patient's trust in her physicians and to encourage her to return to the hospital.

Alternative Views

Other ethical views have been advocated, and it might be objected that one or more of them is preferable to the view I have presented. To further defend my view, let me turn to the main alternatives and the reasons for rejecting them.

One view, advocated by a number of authors, is that coercive treatment of mentally competent obstetric patients is never ethically justifiable.[53] The difficulty with this view is that it constitutes a rigid rule that does not adequately take into account exceptional clinical situations that can occur. An example would be the modified version of the *Jamaica Hospital* case, in which a pregnant woman's refusal of life-saving treatment involves the abandonment of her ten children. In rare cases such as this, there are compelling reasons to override maternal autonomy. Perhaps it will be objected that permitting exceptions to the rule forbidding forced treatment will lead to further invasions of patient autonomy. Some see a potential for enormous regulation of the lives of pregnant women.[54] I agree that regulating the lives of pregnant women is highly undesirable, but it is implausible to believe that the view I have defended would lead to such regulation. Rather, it amounts to a strong barrier against such control of women. It states that interfering with the woman's autonomy is almost never justifiable. From a practical point of view, the position I am defending provides a clear rule of thumb for clinicians — Don't override the competent obstetric patient's autonomy. The burden of proof would be on the clinician to establish that a given case is a truly exceptional one in which there are compelling reasons for intervening. Such reasons usually do not exist. In fact, with the possible exception of the *Jamaica Hospital* case, compelling reasons have been lacking in all of the reported court cases involving forced treatment. The court cases in which placenta previa had been diagnosed involved interventions that were ethically unjustifiable, in part because those particular cases involved a high risk of driving the patient away from medical care.[55] Similarly, the hospital incarcerations of diabetic patients were ethically unjustifiable, involving an excessively high intrusion upon the liberty of pregnant patients.[56] Similar shortcomings can be found in the other reported legal cases. If the view I am advocating had been followed, those forced treatments would not have occurred.

A second view was put forward by the American Medical Association Board of Trustees.[57] According to this view, court-ordered treatment sometimes is ethically justifiable, provided it meets all of the following conditions: (1) it poses insignificant or no health risks for the woman; (2) it involves minimal invasion of the woman's bodily integrity; and (3) it would clearly prevent substantial and irreversible fetal harm. The American Medical Association Board of Trustees did not provide examples of any actual medical procedures that fulfill these conditions; in fact, it is difficult to think of any that do. However, a hypothetical example was provided: Suppose that a drug existed that could be taken orally, would cause no ill effects to the woman, and was needed to prevent substantial harm to the fetus. If the woman refused the medicine, a court would be justified in ordering her to take it, according to the American Medical Association statement. The difficulty with this view is that it also is too inflexible to deal with exceptional situations. Again, the modified version of the *Jamaica Hospital* case illustrates the problem. Because a blood transfusion presumably involves more than a "minimal" invasion of bodily integrity, the American Medical Association position would hold that courts are never justified in ordering a transfusion against the wishes of a competent patient. Yet, the case example suggests that such action sometimes is ethically warranted.

A third view was advocated by the American Academy of Pediatrics Committee on Bioethics.[58] In this view, court-ordered treatment is sometimes justifiable, provided that: (1) the maternal risk posed by the treatment is low; (2) there is a substantial likelihood that the fetus will suffer irrevocable harm without the intervention; and (3) the intervention is clearly appropriate and will likely be effective. Again, no specific examples were given. This view places no restrictions on the invasiveness of the procedure, in contrast to the American Medical Association Board of Trustees' position. However, a main difficulty with this view is that it is inconsistent with the current legal framework, which does not permit interventions involving *any* degree of increased risk, on balance, for the woman. This view also can be criticized on *ethical* grounds because it permits the obstetrician to perform procedures against the woman's wishes that, on balance, increase the risks of physical harm to her. Thus, it violates the principle of doing no harm, as it applies to the woman. In no other area of medicine is it considered ethical for a physician to expose one patient to risks of physical harm against her wishes in order to benefit another patient. Although some might believe that there is an exception to this principle in regard to pregnant patients because they have obligations to their fetuses, this overlooks the arguments supporting a strong presumption against infringing the liberty of pregnant women. The fact that the view in question requires physicians to expose some patients to risks of physical harm for the sake of other patients casts doubt upon its ethical justifiability. Because of the combined legal and ethical difficulties facing the American Academy of Pediatrics' view, it seems reasonable to reject it.

A fourth view has been advocated by Chervenak and McCullough. In an early statement of their position, they claimed that coercive treatment is ethically justifiable if the following conditions hold: (1) the risks to the fetus associated with treatment are minimal; (2) the potential benefit for the fetus is substantial; and (3) the risks to the woman are ones that she should reasonably accept on behalf of the fetus. In other words, they claimed that whenever the woman refuses treatment to which she *ought* to consent, it is ethically justifiable to treat her coercively, provided the other two stated conditions are satisfied.[59]

There are at least two major difficulties with this view. First, as I have stated, it is not obvious that morality ought to be enforced *whenever* the treatment in question would potentially provide a substantial net benefit to the fetal patient. From the fact that a pregnant woman *ought* to do something, it does not automatically follow that forcing her to do it is justifiable. An argument would be needed to defend the view that it is ethically justifiable to enforce morality in the situations in question. Second, the view in question permits the physician to violate the principle of doing no harm with respect to one patient, against her wishes, in order to benefit another patient. To see this, we need only consider that there are situations in which the woman ought to consent, for the sake of the fetus, to procedures that involve a net increase in risk to her.[60] Such action is, on the face of it, a violation of the ethics of the doctor-patient relationship. An argument would be needed to justify such action in this context. However, Chervenak and McCullough do not satisfactorily address these two problems. In the article in which they initially presented their view, these problems are not discussed at all.[61] In a subsequent article, they defend coerced emergency cesarean section without a court order in a case involving a mentally competent woman at thirty-nine weeks' gestation with placental abruption accompanied by persistent fetal bradycardia. However, their argument in this article also fails to address these problems satisfactorily.[62]

Moreover, counterexamples can be given to the view in question. Consider the case described at the beginning of this chapter involving fetal distress, diagnosed on the basis of persistent, clearly documented late decelerations, loss of beat-to-beat variability that did not resolve with less invasive interventions such as repositioning and administration of oxygen, and the appearance of meconium in the amniotic fluid.[63] These clinical findings provided evidence that there was fetal hypoxia and supported a reasonable medical judgment that prompt cesarean delivery was in the interests of the fetus in order to try to prevent brain damage or death. It can be argued that the pregnant woman in this situation had an obligation to agree to cesarean section, based on several considerations: she had a parental duty to protect the well-being of her fetus; that duty was a serious one because the fetus had a relatively high degree of conferred moral standing; the magnitude of potential harm to the fetus was great; the probability of harm to the fetus, although not anywhere near certainty, was high enough that the situation could reasonably be considered a genuine threat to the fetus; and the risks to the woman of cesarean section, while real, were not great enough to exceed the limits of risks that a parent might reasonably be expected to take, given the risks to the fetus of foregoing cesarean section in that situation.

However, forced treatment was not ethically justifiable in that case. A main reason pertains to the *likelihood* that harm would occur to the fetus if cesarean section were not performed. Although the probability of harm was great enough to create an obligation on the part of the woman to consent to cesarean section, it was not great enough to justify forcing her to undergo the surgery. In a significant number of cases, monitor tracings indicating fetal distress are false positives. In other words, although the monitoring indicates fetal distress, the infant's condition after emergency cesarean delivery is not characterized by serious distress.[64] I would suggest that a necessary condition for the ethical justifiability of forced cesarean section is that it be highly likely that surgical delivery would be effective in preventing serious harm to the fetus. Cesarean section is a relatively invasive procedure that involves pain, risks of morbidity, a small but real risk of mortality, and required hospitalization. This indicates that cesarean section against a patient's wishes involves such a significant invasion of bodily integrity that only the most compelling of reasons would justify it. When the likelihood of harm to the fetus without cesarean delivery is below high probability, there are less than fully compelling reasons for forced treatment. Thus, the case being considered undermines the view that morality ought to be enforced whenever treatment during pregnancy potentially would provide a substantial net benefit to the fetal patient.

Another problem with the view of Chervenak and McCullough is its inconsistency with the current legal framework. In particular, it is at odds with the precedent set in the case of A. C. To see this, we need only note that in *many cases* involving treatment refusal by pregnant women, a reasonable argument can be made that the woman morally *ought* to consent to the treatment in question. For example, this is true in many (but not necessarily all) cases involving refusal of cesarean section for competently diagnosed fetal distress, placental abruption, failed progress of labor with prolonged ruptured membranes, placental insufficiency, or complete placenta previa. Thus, the view of Chervenak and McCullough implies that court orders for forced maternal treatment would be justifiable in a substantial percentage of cases involving maternal refusal of treatment. Yet, the precedent of *In re A. C.* states that such court orders should almost never be issued. In addition, the view of Chervenak and McCullough would require the woman to undergo procedures involving a net increase in risks to her, but this is legally inconsistent with the argument based on *Thornburgh*. These inconsistencies with the legal framework make their view impractical because it would often encourage physicians to seek court orders that would be unjustifiable based on the current legal precedents.[65]

Therefore, each of the main alternative views that have been put forward involves serious difficulties and should be rejected.

Epilogue

To conclude, let us return to a statement made in the Introduction and again in Chapter 4. I said that one test of the ethical framework would be its usefulness in resolving ethical issues in reproductive and perinatal medicine. The reader, of course, can be the final judge of whether the framework passes this test. In defense of the framework, I would like to point out several main ways it has proven helpful.

One feature of the framework was an exploration of reasons for valuing freedom to procreate, and a number of such reasons were identified. These reasons were useful when we turned to discussions of donor insemination for single women, ovum donation for "older" women, and surrogate motherhood. For example, in discussing ovum donation for postmenopausal women, I pointed out that a number of the reasons for valuing freedom to procreate are applicable, including the following: procreation involves participation in the creation of a person; it can affirm mutual love; it provides a link to future persons; it involves experiences of pregnancy and childbirth; and it can lead to experiences associated with child rearing. These considerations played a role in the argument that ovum donation for older women sometimes is ethically justifiable. The reasons also were useful in discussing the disposition of pre-embryos; they helped explain why progenitors should have the authority to make decisions concerning the disposition of preembryos and why donation of preembryos to infertile couples is ethically justifiable.

Another aspect of the framework was an exploration of why freedom not to procreate should be valued. These reasons turned out to be useful in discussing the abortion issue, which arose in the context of decision making after detection of fetal anomalies. I argued that freedom not to procreate is important for self-determination, and that self-determination is especially important to women because it is necessary for gaining social equality. These concerns were part of the argument for the ethical justifiability of abortion, together with consideration of the moral status of the fetus. The abortion issue also arose in the context of selective abortion following prenatal testing for "minor" diseases and nondisease characteristics. Self-determination and the importance of nondirective counseling played a role in the argument that it is ethically justifiable to test and abort for "minor" diseases but not nondisease characteristics. The reasons for valuing freedom not to procreate also were pertinent to the disposition of preembryos, in that they helped explain why progenitors should have dispositional authority.

A view concerning the moral status of preembryos, embryos, fetuses, and infants was yet another component of the framework. This view played a central role in discussions of a number of issues. For example, it was applied to issues concerning preembryos, contributing to a defense of research using preembryos and a defense of preimplantation testing for genes causing diseases. It entered into the argument against prenatal testing and abortion for nondisease characteristics. It also was used in discussing the recommendations physicians should make following detection of fetal anomalies, where it played an important role in arguments concerning the justifiability of aggressive and nonaggressive management recommendations in various types of situations. Moreover, it figured into my defense of a view concerning coercive interventions during pregnancy.

Finally, a view concerning how to assign priorities to conflicting ethical values was an important feature of the framework. This view advocating a casuistic approach was directly applicable to all of the issues discussed. It appeared, for example, in the discussion of donor insemination for single women, where I argued that physician compliance with such requests usually is ethically justifiable but sometimes is not. It was used in other contexts where decisions should be based on the presence of various casuistic factors, including the disposition of preembryos following divorce and physician recommendations following detection of fetal anomalies. Also, I argued that the method of assigning priorities should be flexible enough that case-by-case decision making might sometimes be set aside in favor of assigning the same priority to conflicting values in all cases for a given issue. The need for this feature was illustrated by the issues of prenatal and preimplantation genetic testing for enhancement purposes. In addition, I suggested that case-by-case decision making should be flexible enough to incorporate, at least sometimes, a strong presumption in favor of certain values. The need for this feature was illustrated in the discussion of coercive interventions during pregnancy.

All things considered, I believe that the framework proves to be quite useful in the attempt to arrive at reasonable answers to these complex issues.

Notes

Introduction

1. Carl Wood and Alan Trounson, "In-Vitro Fertilization," *Medical Journal of Australia* 146 (1987): 338–40; Karen Dawson, "In Vitro Fertilisation: Legislation and Problems of Research," *British Medical Journal* 295 (1987): 1184–86.

2. Carson Strong, "Justification in Ethics," in Baruch A. Brody, ed., *Moral Theory and Moral Judgments in Medical Ethics* (Dordrecht: Kluwer, 1988), 193–211.

3. James W. Cornman, Keith Lehrer, and George S. Pappas, *Philosophical Problems and Arguments: An Introduction*, 3d ed. (Indianapolis: Hackett, 1987), 315; Bruce Aune, *Kant's Theory of Morals* (Princeton: Princeton University Press, 1979), 191–97.

4. John Robertson, *Children of Choice: Freedom and the New Reproductive Technologies* (Princeton: Princeton University Press, 1994); Laurence B. McCullough and Frank A. Chervenak, *Ethics in Obstetrics and Gynecology* (New York: Oxford University Press, 1994).

5. Also, although McCullough and Chervenak put forward a view concerning the moral status of fetuses, there are difficulties with their view, which I discuss in Chapter 3.

Chapter 1

1. This sterilization law is discussed in *Skinner v. Oklahoma* 316 U.S. 535, 86 L. ed. 1655 (1941).

2. *Stump v. Sparkman* 435 U.S. 349, 55 L. ed. 2d 331 (1978).

3. I follow the customary practice of using the terms *reproduce* and *procreate* interchangeably.

4. For example, in discussing eugenics Francis Crick, codiscoverer of the structure of DNA, stated: " . . . I do not see why people should have the right to have children. I think that if we can get across to people the idea that their children are not entirely their own business and that it is not a private matter, it would be an enormous step forward." Biochemist Norman W. Pirie agreed: "Taking up Crick's point about the humanist argument on whether one has a right to have children, I would say that in a society in which the community is responsible for people's welfare — health, hospitals, unemployment insurance, etc. — the answer is 'No.' " Gordon Wolstenholme, ed., *Man and His Future* (Boston: Little, Brown, 1963), 275, 282.

5. This distinction is noted by John A. Robertson, "Embryos, Families, and Procreative Liberty: The Legal Structure of the New Reproduction," *Southern California Law Review* 59 (1986): 939–1041, 955.

6. John A. Robertson, "Procreative Liberty and the Control of Conception, Pregnancy, and Childbirth," *Virginia Law Review* 69 (1983): 405–64, 408.

7. Robertson, "Procreative Liberty," 410.

8. John A. Robertson, *Children of Choice: Freedom and the New Reproductive Technologies* (Princeton: Princeton University Press, 1994), 22.

9. I do not mean to imply that the expression "having a child of one's own" could not legitimately be given other meanings. Some might argue, for example, that begetting is not a necessary part of "having a child of one's own." Consider an infertile woman who becomes a gestational mother after receiving a donated ovum fertilized with her husband's semen. It might be argued that upon giving birth there is a sense in which she has a child of her own. However, I wish to focus for now on what I take to be the usual meaning of the expression, as defined in the text. My aim is to begin with a form of procreation that is familiar. Any insights gained will then be applied to less familiar modes of procreation; in Chapter 5, for example, I shall consider reproduction involving third-party collaboration.

10. See, e.g., Barbara Eck Menning, "The Emotional Needs of Infertile Couples," *Fertility and Sterility* 34 (1980): 313–19; Miriam D. Mazor, "Emotional Reactions to Infertility" in Miriam D. Mazor and Harriet F. Simons, eds., *Infertility: Medical, Emotional, and Social Considerations* (New York: Human Sciences Press, 1984), 23–35; Judith N. Lasker and Susan Borg, *In Search of Parenthood: Coping with Infertility and High-Tech Conception* (Boston: Beacon, 1987); Machelle M. Seibel and Melvin L. Taymor, "Emotional Aspects of Infertility," *Fertility and Sterility* 37 (1982): 137–45; Deborah P. Valentine, "Psychological Impact of Infertility: Identifying Issues and Needs," *Social Work in Health Care* 11 (1986): 61–69; Patricia P. Mahlstedt, "The Psychological Component of Infertility," *Fertility and Sterility* 43 (1985): 335–46; and Judith C. Daniluk, "Infertility: Intrapersonal and Interpersonal Impact," *Fertility and Sterility* 49 (1988): 982–90.

11. Menning, "Emotional Needs," 314–15; Mazor, "Emotional Reactions," 26; Valentine, "Psychological Impact," 64–65; Mahlstedt, "Psychological Component," 336–41.

12. Menning, "Emotional Needs," 316; Mazor, "Emotional Reactions," 27; Seibel and Taymor, "Emotional Aspects," 138; Mahlstedt, "Psychological Component," 338.

13. Mahlstedt, "Psychological Component," 341.

14. A review of such studies is found in Edward Pohlman, assisted by Julia Mae Pohlman, *The Psychology of Birth Planning* (Cambridge, Mass.: Schenkman, 1969), 35–47.

15. Bill Cosby, *Fatherhood* (Garden City, N.Y.: Doubleday, 1986), 18.

16. Ellen Peck and Judith Senderowitz, eds., *Pronatalism: The Myth of Mom and Apple Pie* (New York: Crowell, 1974). In describing these pressures, Jean E. Veevers states, "In the Western world, there is one expectation about which almost everyone agrees: married couples should have children. Moreover, it is not enough that couples have children: they are also expected to want to have them. Parenthood is almost universally lauded as an intrinsically desirable social role." See Veevers, *Childless by Choice* (Toronto: Butterworths, 1980), 1.

17. Veevers, *Childless by Choice*, 5–6.

18. Lee Rainwater was one of the first researchers to document negative attitudes toward persons who do not have children. In a study of 96 men and women, he found that childlessness met with disapproval. See Rainwater, assisted by K. K. Weinstein, *And the Poor Get Children* (Chicago: Quadrangle, 1960). Janet Griffith surveyed a large sample of married couples and asked them to imagine that they were childless. Three-fourths of them stated that parents or other close relatives would urge them to have a child, and two-thirds stated that close friends would. Nearly half believed that others would regard them as selfish. See Griffith, "Social Pressures on Family Size Intentions," *Family Planning Perspectives* 5 (1973): 237–42. Denise F. Polit surveyed randomly selected subjects and found that the voluntarily childless were stereotyped as "more socially undesirable, less well adjusted, less nurturant, more autonomous, more succorant, and more socially distant than individuals of other fertility statuses." See Polit, "Stereotypes Relating to Family Size Status," *Journal of Marriage and the Family* 40 (1978): 105–14.

19. Lasker and Borg, *In Search of Parenthood*, 14–17.

20. Judith Blake, "Coercive Pronatalism and American Population Policy," in Peck and Senderowitz, *Pronatalism*, 29–67.

21. Nancy Felipe Russo, "The Motherhood Mandate," *Journal of Social Issues* 32 (1976): 143–53, 143.

22. See, e.g., Christine Overall, *Ethics and Human Reproduction: A Feminist Analysis* (Boston: Allen & Unwin, 1987), 150; Robyn Rowland, "Of Women Born, but for How Long? The Relationship of Women to the New Reproductive Technologies and the Issue of Choice" in Patricia Spallone and Deborah Lynn Steinberg, eds., *Made to Order: The Myth of Reproductive and Genetic Progress* (Oxford: Pergamon, 1987), 67–83; Anne Donchin, "The Growing Feminist Debate over the New Reproductive Technologies," *Hypatia* 4 (1989): 136–49.

23. Michael D. Bayles, *Reproductive Ethics* (Englewood Cliffs: Prentice-Hall, 1984), 3–5, 12–14.

24. Ibid., 13.

25. See Blake, "Coercive Pronatalism," 45–49; Norma Juliet Wikler, "Society's Response to the New Reproductive Technologies: The Feminist Perspectives," *Southern California Law Review* 59 (1986): 1043–57, 1049; Veevers, *Childless by Choice*, 150–51; Sarah Franklin and Maureen McNeil, "Reproductive Futures: Recent Literature and Current Feminist Debates on Reproductive Technologies," *Feminist Studies* 14 (1988): 545–60, 553.

26. Frances Myrna Kamm, review of Bayles, *Reproductive Ethics* in *Canadian Philosophical Review* 5 (1985): 168–73.

27. See, e.g., Pohlman, *Psychology of Birth Planning,* 48–81; Edward Pohlman, "Motivations in Wanting Conceptions" in Peck and Senderowitz, *Pronatalism,* 159–190; Jean E. Veevers, "The Social Meanings of Parenthood," *Psychiatry* 36 (1973): 291–310; Fred Arnold et al., *The Value of Children: A Cross-National Study* (Honolulu: East-West Population Institute, 1975); Eulah Croson Laucks, *The Meaning of Children: Attitudes and Opinions of a Selected Group of U.S. University Graduates* (Boulder: Westview, 1981); and Robert E. Gould, "The Wrong Reasons to Have Children," in Peck and Senderowitz, *Pronatalism,* 193–98.

28. Joseph Ellin, "Sterilization, Privacy, and the Value of Reproduction," in John W. Davis, Barry Hoffmaster, and Sarah Shorter, eds., *Contemporary Issues in Biomedical Ethics* (Clifton, N.J.: Humana, 1978), 114.

29. Jeffrey H. Reiman, "Privacy, Intimacy, and Personhood," *Philosophy and Public Affairs* 6 (1976): 26–44, 33.

30. Ibid., 34–35.

31. See, e.g., Richard A. McCormick, *How Brave a New World? Dilemmas in Bioethics* (Washington, D.C.: Georgetown University Press, 1981), 306–35; and Karl Rahner, "The Problem of Genetic Manipulation," *Theological Investigations,* vol. 9: *Writings of 1965–67,* trans. Graham Harrison (New York: Herder and Herder, 1972), 246.

32. Arthur J. Dyck, "Procreative Rights and Population Policy," *Hastings Center Studies* 1 (1973): 74–82, 75.

33. Marshall Missner, "Why Have Children?" *International Journal of Applied Philosophy* 3 (1987): 1–13, 4.

34. Plato *Symposium* 208d–209e.

35. Cosby, *Fatherhood,* 15.

36. Joel Feinberg, "The Nature and Value of Rights," *Journal of Value Inquiry* 4 (1970): 243–57; and *Social Philosophy* (Englewood Cliffs: Prentice Hall, 1973), 64–67.

37. See, e.g., Richard Wasserstrom, "Rights, Human Rights, and Racial Discrimination," *Journal of Philosophy* 61 (1964): 628–41; and Ronald Dworkin, *Taking Rights Seriously* (Cambridge, Mass.: Harvard University Press, 1977), 184–205.

38. See, e.g., Peter Singer and Deane Wells, *Making Babies: The New Science and Ethics of Conception* (New York: Scribner, 1985), 46–52; and Suzanne Uniacke, "*In Vitro* Fertilization and the Right to Reproduce," *Bioethics* 1 (1987): 241–54.

39. Leon R. Kass, *Toward a More Natural Science: Biology and Human Affairs* (New York: Free Press, 1985), 44.

40. See, e.g., Susan Rae Peterson, "The Politics of Prenatal Diagnosis: A Feminist Ethical Analysis," in Helen B. Holmes, Betty B. Hoskins, and Michael Gross, eds., *The Custom-Made Child? Women-Centered Perspectives* (Clifton, N.J.: Humana, 1981), 95–104.

41. For similar accounts of moral rights as closely aligned with the Kantian concept of respect for persons, see, e. g., Feinberg, *Social Philosophy,* 84–94; Dworkin, *Taking Rights Seriously,* 198–99; and Charles Fried, *Right and Wrong* (Cambridge, Mass.: Harvard University Press, 1978). Some might argue that rights can be justified by theories that are not deontological, such as contractarianism or utilitarianism. Even if such justifi-

cation is possible, it does not remove the close relationship between rights and the Kantian concept of human dignity.

42. To my knowledge, no one was ever sterilized under the Oklahoma statute. In *Skinner v. Oklahoma,* the U.S. Supreme Court declared the statute unconstitutional, stating that "we are dealing here with legislation which involves one of the basic civil rights of man. Marriage and procreation are fundamental to the very existence and survival of the race." 316 U.S. 535, at 541. Concerning the Spitler case, in federal court Linda and her husband sued her mother, her mother's attorney, the doctors, the hospital, and Judge Stump, alleging violations of her constitutional rights. The case went to the U.S. Supreme Court, which decided in favor of the defendants. The Court held that arguments based on constitutionality could be made only against the judge, since he was the only state agent in the case. Moreover, the Court ruled that the judge was immune from suit under the doctrine of judicial immunity. The facts of the case are reported in *Stump v. Sparkman* 435 U.S. 349 (1978). The issue of whether nonvoluntary sterilization of mentally retarded persons is ever ethically justifiable is beyond the scope of this chapter.

43. It is worth emphasizing the limited nature of this conclusion. I have argued only that there is a right to procreate in the sense of "having a child" or "having children." Whether there is a right to procreate in other senses, such as being a gamete donor or surrogate mother, remains to be considered.

44. Milton Meltzer, *The Human Rights Book* (New York: Farrar, Straus, and Giroux, 1979), 172–78, 175.

45. Ruth F. Chadwick, ed., *Ethics, Reproduction, and Genetic Control* (London: Croom Helm, 1987), 4.

46. I refer specifically to arrangements in which the ova are provided by the infertile woman, not by the surrogate mother. Such arrangements fit the definition of "having children" stated in the text.

Chapter 2

1. Catherine G. Roraback, "*Griswold v. Connecticut:* A Brief Case History," *Ohio Northern University Law Review* 16 (1989): 395–401.

2. In Chapter 1, I argued that procreating includes raising children one has begotten or gestated. It follows that freedom not to procreate includes freedom not to raise children one has begotten or gestated. However, it should not be assumed that if persons should be free not to beget or gestate, then they should be equally free to avoid raising children they have begotten or gestated. There can be parental obligations toward existing children that place significant limits on freedom not to raise them. In this chapter, I focus on freedom not to beget and freedom not to gestate because they are especially relevant to ethical issues in reproductive and perinatal medicine. The many issues pertaining to avoiding raising one's children are not discussed in this book.

3. *Griswold v. Connecticut* 381 U.S. 479, 14 L. ed. 2d 510 (1965).

4. Ibid., 516.

5. The question of which rights should be regarded as fundamental is discussed by, e.g., David A. J. Richards, "Constitutional Legitimacy and Constitutional Privacy," *New York University Law Review* 61 (1986): 800–862.

6. *Meyer v. Nebraska* 262 U.S. 390, 67 L. ed. 1042 (1923). The Court affirmed the right of parents to direct the upbringing and education of their children in *Pierce v. Society of Sisters* 268 U.S. 510, 69 L. ed. 1070 (1924). This right can be considered a *procreative* right, based on my argument in Chapter 1 that procreation includes rearing children one has begotten or gestated.

7. *Eisenstadt v. Baird* 405 U.S. 438, 31 L. ed. 2d 349 (1972).

8. *Loving v. Virginia* 388 U.S. 1, 18 L. ed. 2d 1010 (1967).

9. *Stanley v. Illinois* 405 U.S. 645, 31 L. ed. 2d 551 (1972).

10. *Roe v. Wade* 410 U.S. 113, 35 L. ed. 2d 147 (1973).

11. *Meyer* 262 U.S. 390, 399.

12. *Roe* 35 L. ed. 2d 147, 177.

13. See, e.g., *Planned Parenthood v. Danforth* 428 U.S. 52 (1976); *Carey v. Population Services* 431 U.S. 678 (1977); *City of Akron v. Akron Center for Reproductive Health* 462 U.S. 416 (1983); *Thornburgh v. American College of Obstetricians and Gynecologists* 476 U.S. 747 (1986); *Webster v. Reproductive Health Services* 492 U.S. 490 (1989); and *Planned Parenthood of Southeastern Pennsylvania v. Casey* 112 S.Ct. 2791, 120 L. ed. 2d 674 (1992).

14. *Casey* 120 L. ed. 2d 674 (1992).

15. Ibid., 714.

16. This new standard constituted a rejection of *Roe*'s trimester framework for deciding when restrictions would be constitutional. See *Casey* 120 L. ed. 2d 674, 712 (1992).

17. See, e.g., Elizabeth L. Beardsley, "Privacy: Autonomy and Selective Disclosure" in J. Roland Pennock and John W. Chapman, eds., *Nomos XIII: Privacy* (New York: Atherton, 1971), 56–70; Judith Jarvis Thomson, "The Right to Privacy,' *Philosophy and Public Affairs* 4 (1975): 295–314; H. J. McCloskey, "Privacy and the Right to Privacy," *Philosophy* 55 (1980): 17–38; W. A. Parent, "Privacy, Morality, and the Law," *Philosophy and Public Affairs* 12 (1983): 269–88; and Parent, "Recent Work on the Concept of Privacy," *American Philosophical Quarterly* 20 (1983): 341–55.

18. Beardsley, "Privacy," 56.

19. Parent, "Privacy, Morality," 269. Parent defines personal information as follows: "Personal information consists of facts which most persons in a given society choose not to reveal about themselves (except to close friends, family . . .) or of facts about which a particular individual is acutely sensitive and which he therefore does not choose to reveal about himself, even though most people don't care if these same facts are widely known about themselves" (270).

20. Parent, "Recent Work," 350.

21. *Griswold* 14 L.ed. 2d 510, 516.

22. See, e.g., John Hart Ely, "The Wages of Crying Wolf: A Comment on *Roe v. Wade*," *Yale Law Journal* 82 (1973): 920–49; Louis Henkin, "Privacy and Autonomy," *Columbia Law Review* 74 (1974): 1410–33; Kent Greenawalt, "Privacy and Its Legal Protections," *Hastings Center Studies* 2 (1974): 45–68; Richard A. Posner, "The Uncertain Protection of Privacy by the Supreme Court," *Supreme Court Review* (1979): 173–216; Thomas Huff, "Thinking Clearly about Privacy," *Washington Law Review* 55 (1980): 777–94; and Parent, "Privacy, Morality," 283–84.

23. *Roe* 35 L. ed. 2d 147, 177.

24. *Casey* 120 L. ed. 2d 674 (1992).

25. See, e.g., Ely, "Wages of Crying Wolf"; Henkin, "Privacy and Autonomy"; Richards, "Constitutional Legitimacy"; Jed Rubenfeld, "The Right of Privacy," *Harvard Law Review* 102 (1989): 737–807; and G. Sidney Buchanan, "The Right of Privacy: Past, Present, and Future," *Ohio Northern University Law Review* 16 (1989): 403–510.

26. David A. J. Richards, "Sexual Autonomy and the Constitutional Right to Privacy: A Case Study in Human Rights and the Unwritten Constitution," *Hastings Law Journal* 30 (1979): 957–1018, 1000, footnotes deleted.

27. Elinor B. Rosenberg, *The Adoption Life Cycle: The Children and Their Families through the Years* (New York: Free Press, 1992), 25–26.

28. See, e.g., Rosenberg, *Adoption Life Cycle*, 26–27; Anthony N. Maluccio, "Casework with Parents of Children in Foster Care" in Paula A. Sinanoglu and Anthony N. Maluccio, eds., *Parents of Children in Placement: Perspectives and Programs* (New York: Child Welfare League of America, 1981), 15–25, 17.

29. Shulamith Firestone, *The Dialectic of Sex: The Case for Feminist Revolution* (New York: Morrow, 1970), 8–9.

30. See, e.g., Christine Overall, *Ethics and Human Reproduction: A Feminist Analysis* (Boston: Allen & Unwin, 1987), 10; Hilary Rose and Jalna Hanmer, "Women's Liberation, Reproduction, and the Technological Fix" in Diana Leonard Barker and Sheila Allen, eds., *Sexual Divisions and Society: Process and Change* (London: Tavistock, 1976), 199–223; Robyn Rowland, "Of Women Born, but for How Long? The Relationship of Women to the New Reproductive Technologies and the Issue of Choice" in Patricia Spallone and Deborah Lynn Steinberg, eds., *Made to Order: The Myth of Reproductive and Genetic Progress* (Oxford: Pergamon, 1987), 67–83;

31. Adrienne Rich, *Of Woman Born: Motherhood as Experience and Institution* (New York: Norton, 1976), 13, 369; Mary O'Brien, *The Politics of Reproduction* (Boston: Routledge & Kegan Paul, 1981), 9–11, 78–82; Laura M. Purdy, "Surrogate Mothering: Exploitation or Empowerment?" *Bioethics* 3 (1989): 18–34; and Rowland, "Of Women Born, but for How Long?" 67–83.

32. Resolution from the FINRRAGE Conference, July 3–8, 1985, Vällinge, Sweden; cited in Spallone and Steinberg, *Made to Order*, 211–12.

33. Alison M. Jaggar and Paula Rothenberg Struhl, *Feminist Frameworks: Alternative Theoretical Accounts of the Relations between Women and Men* (New York: McGraw-Hill, 1978), Introduction, ix–xiv.

34. For further discussion of main types of feminism, see Rosemarie Tong, *Feminist Thought: A Comprehensive Introduction* (Boulder, Colo.: Westview, 1989).

35. See, e.g., Gena Corea, *The Mother Machine: Reproductive Technologies from Artificial Insemination to Artificial Wombs* (New York: Harper & Row, 1985); Ruth Hubbard, "The Case against In Vitro Fertilization and Implantation" in Helen B. Holmes, Betty B. Hoskins, and Michael Gross, eds., *The Custom-Made Child? Women-Centered Perspectives* (Clifton, N.J.: Humana, 1981), 259–62; Maria Mies, "Why Do We Need All This? A Call against Genetic Engineering and Reproductive Technology" in Spallone and Steinberg, *Made to Order*, 34–47; Rowland, "Of Women Born, but for How Long?" 67–83.

36. See, e.g., Lynn M. Paltrow, book review, "Test-Tube Women: What Future for

Motherhood?" *Women's Rights Law Reporter* 8 (1985): 303–7; Rosalind Pollack Petchesky, "Artificial Insemination, In-Vitro Fertilization and the Stigma of Infertility" in Michelle Stanworth, ed., *Reproductive Technologies: Gender, Motherhood and Medicine* (Minneapolis: University of Minnesota Press, 1987), 57–80; Lori B. Andrews, "Alternative Modes of Reproduction" in Sherrill Cohen and Nadine Taub, eds., *Reproductive Laws for the 1990s* (Clifton, N.J.: Humana, 1989), 361–403; Judith N. Lasker and Susan Borg, *In Search of Parenthood: Coping with Infertility and High-Tech Conception* (Boston: Beacon, 1987), 190; Barbara Menning, "In Defense of In Vitro Fertilization" in Holmes, Hoskins, and Gross, *Custom-Made Child,* 263–68; and Mary Anne Warren, "IVF and Women's Interests: An Analysis of Feminist Concerns," *Bioethics* 2 (1988): 37–57.

37. Wendy Chavkin, Barbara Katz Rothman, and Rayna Rapp, "Alternative Modes of Reproduction: Other Views and Questions" in Cohen and Taub, *Reproductive Laws,* 405–9.

38. Lori B. Andrews, "Surrogate Motherhood: The Challenge for Feminists" in Larry Gostin, ed., *Surrogate Motherhood: Politics and Privacy* (Bloomington: Indiana University Press, 1990), 167–82.

39. Overall, *Ethics and Human Reproduction,* 1–16; Andrews, "Alternative Modes," 405–9; Susan Sherwin, "Feminist and Medical Ethics: Two Different Approaches to Contextual Ethics," *Hypatia* 4 (1989): 57–72.

Chapter 3

1. See, e.g., Francoise Laborie, "Looking for Mothers, You Only Find Fetuses" in Patricia Spallone and Deborah Lynn Steinberg, eds., *Made to Order: The Myth of Reproductive and Genetic Progress* (Oxford: Pergamon, 1987), 48–57; Janice C. Raymond, "Fetalists and Feminists: They Are Not the Same" in Spallone and Steinberg, *Made to Order,* 58–66.

2. M. E. Winston, "Abortion and Parental Responsibility," *Journal of Medical Humanities and Bioethics* 7 (1986): 33–56.

3. Norman C. Gillespie, "Abortion and Human Rights," *Ethics* 87 (1977): 237–43, at 238.

4. Michael Tooley has defended this view in the following: "Abortion and Infanticide," *Philosophy and Public Affairs* 2 (1972): 37–65, repr. in Marshall Cohen, Thomas Nagel, and Thomas Scanlon, eds., *The Rights and Wrongs of Abortion* (Princeton: Princeton University Press, 1974), 52–84; "In Defense of Abortion and Infanticide" in Joel Feinberg, ed., *The Problem of Abortion,* 2d ed. (Belmont, Cal.: Wadsworth, 1984), 120–34; and *Abortion and Infanticide* (Oxford: Oxford University Press, 1983). The quotation is from "Abortion and Infanticide," 59.

5. President's Commission for the Study of Ethical Problems in Medicine and Biomedical and Behavioral Research, *Deciding to Forgo Life-Sustaining Treatment* (Washington, D.C.: Government Printing Office, 1983), 197–229; Arthur Caplan and Cynthia B. Cohen, eds., "Imperiled Newborns," *Hastings Center Report* 17 (1987): 5–32.

6. Loren E. Lomasky, "Being a Person—Does It Matter?" *Philosophical Topics* 12 (1982), repr. in Feinberg, *Problem of Abortion,* 161–72, at 169.

7. Philip E. Devine, *The Ethics of Homicide* (Ithaca: Cornell University Press, 1978), 94.

8. H. Tristram Engelhardt, Jr., *The Foundations of Bioethics* (New York: Oxford University Press, 1986), 111.

9. Bonnie Steinbock, *Life before Birth: The Moral and Legal Status of Embryos and Fetuses* (New York: Oxford University Press, 1992), 59.

10. Helga Kuhse and Peter Singer, "The Moral Status of the Embryo: Two Viewpoints" in William Walters and Peter Singer, eds., *Test-Tube Babies* (Melbourne: Oxford University Press, 1982), 57–63.

11. Stephen Buckle, "Arguing from Potential," *Bioethics* 2 (1988): 227–53.

12. Ibid., 233–34, 237.

13. As Buckle puts it: "If allowing a present embryo to develop will produce a future state that is less valuable than preventing the development of this embryo, and developing instead another, not yet conceived, embryo (for example, if the present one is suffering from a congenital defect, or if the parents or other appropriately placed parties are unable to care adequately for it), then a straightforward application of consequentialist principles requires that we follow the latter course." Ibid., 242.

14. Ibid., 238–39.

15. Devine, *Ethics of Homicide*, 74, 94.

16. Ibid., 95.

17. Leonard Glantz's example is presented in George Annas, "A French Homunculus in a Tennessee Court," *Hastings Center Report* 19 (1989): 20–22.

18. Ethics Committee of the American Fertility Society, "Ethical Considerations of the New Reproductive Technologies," *Fertility and Sterility* 53, suppl. 2 (1990): i–vii, 1S–104S, at vii.

19. L. W. Sumner, *Abortion and Moral Theory* (Princeton: Princeton University Press, 1981).

20. Ibid., 143–44.

21. Ibid., 152.

22. Joel Feinberg, "The Rights of Animals and Unborn Generations" in William T. Blackstone, ed., *Philosophy and Environmental Crisis* (Athens, Ga.: University of Georgia Press, 1974), 43–68, at 52.

23. *Roe v. Wade,* 35 L. ed. 2d 181.

24. Norman Fost, David Chudwin, and Daniel Wikler, "The Limited Moral Significance of Fetal Viability," *Hastings Center Report* 10 (1980): 10–13, at 13.

25. Devine, *Ethics of Homicide,* 86.

26. Roger Wertheimer, "Understanding the Abortion Argument," *Philosophy and Public Affairs* 1 (1971): 67–95, at 82.

27. Alan Zaitchik, "Viability and the Morality of Abortion," *Philosophy and Public Affairs* 10 (1980): 18–26.

28. Nancy Rhoden has given a similar explanation of why the viability criterion might be appealing. She distinguishes between viability as technological survivability and viability as a normative concept. On her view, normative viability has at least two major components: technological survivability and a degree of development so substantial that the fetus has a claim to societal protection. She suggests that the reason the viability criterion seemed plausible to the Supreme Court is that in 1973 viability clearly coincided

with late gestation. See Nancy Rhoden, "Trimesters and Technology: Revamping *Roe V. Wade,*" *Yale Law Journal* 95 (1986): 639–97, at 643, 658, 671–72.

29. Laurence B. McCullough and Frank A. Chervenak, *Ethics in Obstetrics and Gynecology* (New York: Oxford University Press, 1994), 96–110; Frank A. Chervenak and Laurence B. McCullough, "Does Obstetric Ethics Have Any Role in the Obstetrician's Response to the Abortion Controversy?" *American Journal of Obstetrics and Gynecology* 163 (1990): 1425–29.

30. McCullough and Chervenak, *Ethics in Obstetrics and Gynecology,* 97.

31. Ibid., 104.

32. Ibid., 102.

33. Ibid., 104.

34. McCullough and Chervenak refer to this moral status as *dependent* because it is based on factors other than the inherent characteristics of the fetus.

35. Steinbock, *Life before Birth,* 53–54.

36. A number of commentators have made the distinction between *intrinsic* and *conferred* moral standing, although this particular terminology is not uniformly used. Engelhardt, for example, argues that individuals who possess self-consciousness, rationality, and a minimal moral sense (an understanding of the notion of worthiness of blame and praise) have full moral standing because of their intrinsic characteristics, and he refers to such individuals as persons in the strict sense. He also argues that it is morally justifiable to confer significant moral status on certain types of individuals who lack what I am calling descriptive personhood, and he refers to this status as being a person for social considerations. See Engelhardt, *Foundations of Bioethics,* 104–9, 116. Similarly, Roger Wertheimer uses the terms *independent* and *dependent* moral status to denote what is essentially the same distinction as that between intrinsic and conferred standing; see "Philosophy on Humanity" in Robert L. Perkins, ed., *Abortion: Pro and Con* (Cambridge, Mass.: Schenkman, 1974), 107–28. Ronald M. Green makes a similar distinction using a contractarian approach. He argues that fundamental rights are possessed by individuals who are capable of participating in a contractarian choice procedure. According to Green, infants and fetuses might have some degree of moral standing conferred on them, even though they themselves are incapable of participating in the choice procedure. See Ronald M. Green, "Conferred Rights and the Fetus," *Journal of Religious Ethics* 2 (1974): 55–75.

37. S. I. Benn, "Abortion, Infanticide, and Respect for Persons" in Feinberg, *Problem of Abortion,* 135–44, at 143.

38. Ibid.

39. Joel Feinberg, "Potentiality, Development, and Rights" in ibid., 145–50, at 149.

40. Feinberg, "Potentiality, Development," 150.

41. In Engelhardt's words, the level of interaction between mother and child is different in kind from the level of interaction between mother and fetus. The first is actually and explicitly social; the second is primarily biological and occurs automatically without active involvement of the mother, See H. Tristram Engelhardt, Jr., "Viability, Abortion, and the Difference between a Fetus and an Infant," *American Journal of Obstetrics and Gynecology* 116 (1973): 429–34, at 432. More recently, Engelhardt has qualified his view, claiming that the argument for conferred moral status is less strong during the

neonatal period than it is later when the child is more fully socialized. See Engelhardt, *Foundations of Bioethics,* 116, 119.

42. Engelhardt, *Foundations of Bioethics,* 117.

43. Mary Anne Warren, "The Moral Significance of Birth," *Hypatia* 4 (1989): 46–65, at 56–57.

44. Green, "Conferred Rights," 59.

45. Ibid., 63.

46. Jane English, "Abortion and the Concept of a Person," *Canadian Journal of Philosophy* 5 (1975): 233–43, at 241.

47. In this section I attempt to develop and defend more fully a view on moral standing which I stated in "Delivering Hydrocephalic Fetuses," *Bioethics* 5 (1991): 1–22; see also Carson Strong and Garland D. Anderson, "An Ethical Framework for Issues during Pregnancy" in Raanan Gillon, ed., *Principles of Health Care Ethics* (Chichester: Wiley, 1994), 587–600.

48. Strong, "Delivering Hydrocephalic Fetuses," 11.

49. K. J. S. Anand and P. R. Hickey, "Pain and Its Effects in the Human Neonate and Fetus," *New England Journal of Medicine* 317 (1987): 1321–29.

50. Warren, "Moral Significance of Birth," 59.

51. This point is discussed further in Chapter 4 below, in the section on utilitarianism. See also Carson Strong, "Justification in Ethics" in Baruch A. Brody, ed., *Moral Theory and Moral Judgments in Medical Ethics* (Dordrecht: Kluwer, 1988), 193–211.

52. Winston, "Abortion and Parental Responsibility."

53. Deborah Mathieu, "Respecting Liberty and Preventing Harm: Limits of State Intervention in Prenatal Choice," *Harvard Journal of Law and Public Policy* 8 (1985): 19–55, 37.

Chapter 4

1. These principles are discussed more fully in Tom L. Beauchamp and James F. Childress, *Principles of Biomedical Ethics,* 4th ed. (New York: Oxford University Press, 1994). K. Danner Clouser and Bernard Gert refer to these principles as the mantra of bioethics, but argue that middle-level principles alone do not provide an adequate moral framework for bioethics. See Clouser and Gert, "A Critique of Principlism," *Journal of Medicine and Philosophy* 15 (1990): 219–36.

2. For discussions of an ethical framework based on moral rules, see Bernard Gert, *The Moral Rules* (New York: Harper and Row, 1970); and *Morality: A New Justification of the Moral Rules* (New York: Oxford University Press, 1988). Ethical values also include the concerns expressed by maxims, as that term is used by Albert R. Jonsen and Stephen Toulmin in their discussions of casuistic reasoning in ethics. They use the term *maxim* to refer both to moral principles and rules. See Jonsen and Toulmin, *The Abuse of Casuistry* (Berkeley: University of California Press, 1988), 252–53.

3. Baruch A. Brody, *Life and Death Decision Making* (New York: Oxford University Press, 1988), 33.

4. The resolution of issues in Part 2 generally will not hinge on which version of consequentialism we use. Therefore, I shall remain neutral between them.

5. See Chap. 3 above.

6. Duties often can be thought of as counterparts to rights. Some hold that for every duty there is a corresponding right, while others maintain that it makes sense to speak of duties to oneself, for which there are no corresponding rights. This is an issue we need not settle here.

7. These and other virtues relevant to health care are discussed by Brody in *Life and Death Decision Making*, 35–42. See also Laurence B. McCullough and Frank A. Chervenak, *Ethics in Obstetrics and Gynecology* (New York: Oxford University Press, 1994), 82–87.

8. Carol Gilligan, *In a Different Voice: Psychological Theory and Women's Development* (Cambridge, Mass.: Harvard University Press, 1982). See also Eric H. Loewy, "Care Ethics: A Concept in Search of a Framework," *Cambridge Quarterly of Healthcare Ethics* 4 (1995): 56–63.

9. Part of this section is adapted from Carson Strong, "Justification in Ethics" in Baruch A. Brody, ed., *Moral Theory and Moral Judgments in Medical Ethics* (Dordrecht: Kluwer, 1988), 193–211.

10. According to utilitarianism, the only relevant consideration in assessing the rightness of our actions is the good and bad consequences that we bring about. On this view, we should strive to maximize good consequences, or *utility*. Utilitarianism holds that the good of each person is to count equally and that we should strive to bring about the greatest good for the greatest number. Two formulations of utilitarianism can be distinguished, depending on whether one chooses *rules* of behavior that maximize utility or specific *acts* that maximize it.

11. It might be objected that the difficulty in making defensible predictions is due to our current state of ignorance and that if we wished, we could carry out psychosocial research to obtain the necessary data. Because utilitarianism is correct, it might be argued, this is precisely what we should do. However, this objection overlooks serious problems concerning both the ethics and the scientific design of studies that would provide such data. In "Justification in Ethics," 196–97, I respond to this objection and argue that it is unreasonable to believe that the necessary data can be obtained. It might also be objected that cost-effectiveness and cost-benefit analyses sometimes are applied to policy issues in medicine, thereby suggesting that utilitarian reasoning can give practical guidance. Cost-effectiveness analysis does not consider good and bad consequences that are nonmonetary. Therefore, it has serious limitations and is not truly a form of utilitarianism, which requires consideration of *all* relevant consequences. By contrast, cost-benefit analysis can be considered truly utilitarian but faces serious conceptual problems. First, there is the problem of satisfactorily quantifying on a single scale seemingly disparate good and bad consequences, such as prevention of pain, promotion of truth telling, loss of life, and invasion of privacy. Second, there is the problem of making defensible predictions, which I discussed above.

12. Immanuel Kant, *Foundations of the Metaphysics of Morals,* trans. Lewis White Beck (Indianapolis: Bobbs-Merrill, 1959), 47.

13. In Chap. 3, I argued for conferring the status of normative personhood upon infants. Thus, infants and other children should be treated as ends in themselves.

14. For Kant, all moral duties can be divided into two categories: duties of justice and duties of virtue. In part one of *The Metaphysics of Morals* he discusses duties of justice. He attempts to show how these duties can be derived from the categorical imperative by means of an intermediate principle called the Universal Law of Justice, which is stated as follows: Act externally in such a way that the free use of your will is compatible with the freedom of everyone according to a universal law. Part 1 is published as *The Metaphysical Elements of Justice*, trans. John Ladd (Indianapolis: Bobbs-Merrill, 1965); quotation from p. 35. In part 2 Kant discusses duties of virtue. He tries to show how these duties can be derived from the categorical imperative using an intermediate principle called the Universal Ethical Command, stated as: Act dutifully from a sense of duty. Part 2 is published as *The Metaphysical Principles of Virtue*, trans. James Ellington (Indianapolis: Bobbs-Merrill, 1964); quotation from p. 49.

15. Kant holds that there can be no conflicting obligations. However, this view arises because he uses the terms *obligation* and *duty* to refer to *necessary* duties (or what we might call *all things considered* duties), as opposed to prima facie duties. Yet, he recognizes that there are situations in which different actions are required by different rules (*maxims*, to use his term). In such cases the conflicting maxims constitute conflicting *grounds of obligation*. In modern terms we would say that in such cases there are conflicting prima facie duties. See *The Metaphysical Principles of Virtue*, 24.

16. Kant seems to acknowledge in *The Metaphysics of Morals* that his theoretical framework is not capable, as it stands, of resolving conflicts in particular cases. This is pointed out by Bruce Aune, who states the following:

> Kant's failure to provide clear directions for resolving conflicts between various grounds of obligation is perhaps explained by a remark he makes toward the end of his Ethical Doctrine of Elements, which is the principle section of his Doctrine of Virtue. The remark is that the duties of men to one another with regard to their *circumstances* do not call for a special chapter in a system of pure ethics; they can be specified only by the application of pure principles to experience. To deal with the full range of moral problems that arise for us, we thus need, he says, a transition from pure to applied ethics — one that, by applying the pure principles of duty to cases of experience, would *schematize* these principles, as it were, and present them as ready for morally-practical use. Without such a transition, we shall not have, he adds, a complete exposition of our system of ethics. Unfortunately, he does not include such a transition in his Doctrine of Virtue.

See Bruce Aune, *Kant's Theory of Morals* (Princeton: Princeton University Press, 1979), 193, references deleted. Aune provides a helpful discussion of the inability of Kant's theory to resolve conflicting duties in particular cases: see esp. pp. 191–97.

17. Onora Nell has suggested that conflicts of duty might be resolved using Kant's first formulation of the categorical imperative: Act only on the maxim through which you can at the same time will that it should become a universal law. However, Nell acknowledges that her proposed method works only in those cases in which it is clear which duty should be given priority, and is not very helpful in difficult cases. Unfortunately, the conflicts of duties we face in reproductive and perinatal medicine tend to be difficult ones in which

there is lack of clarity and consensus about what should be done. Thus, Nell's proposal does not provide the guidance we seek. See Onora Nell, *Acting on Principle: An Essay on Kantian Ethics* (New York: Columbia University Press, 1975), 132–37.

18. John Rawls, *A Theory of Justice* (Cambridge: Harvard University Press, 1971).

19. Robert M. Veatch, *A Theory of Medical Ethics* (New York: Basic Books, 1981).

20. Veatch, *Theory of Medical Ethics,* 298–303, 328. In a *lexical* ordering, ethical values are ordered hierarchically, giving some value or set of values priority over all others. Another value or set of values is ranked second, taking priority over all except those ranked first, and so on. One may not act to promote a lower-ranked value in any situation unless there is no conflict with higher-ranked values.

21. Ibid., 304.

22. Ibid.

23. Ibid., 298–303.

24. Joseph Fletcher, *The Ethics of Genetic Control* (Buffalo: Prometheus, 1988).

25. An argument Veatch gives for the view that autonomy always overrides beneficence is that the exceptionless right of mentally competent patients to refuse to participate in medical research only makes sense if autonomy has absolute priority over beneficence. If we allow the possibility that beneficence sometimes outweighs autonomy, he suggests, then we must be committed to the view that conscripting competent subjects for research without their informed consent would be acceptable provided the potential benefits of the research were great enough. See Robert M. Veatch, "Resolving Conflicts among Principles: Ranking, Balancing, and Specifying," *Kennedy Institute of Ethics Journal* 5 (1995): 199–218. However, Veatch's conclusion does not follow. One can hold that beneficence overrides autonomy in some types of cases — e.g., preventing harm to innocent third parties — while also holding that beneficence does not override autonomy in other types of cases, such as those raising the question of whether competent subjects may be conscripted for research without informed consent.

26. This third approach is discussed in Terrence F. Ackerman and Carson Strong, *A Casebook of Medical Ethics* (New York: Oxford University Press, 1989), where it is referred to as the balancing approach.

27. Jonsen and Toulmin, *Abuse of Casuistry.* See also Albert R. Jonsen, "On Being a Casuist" in Terrence F. Ackerman et al., eds., *Clinical Medical Ethics: Exploration and Assessment* (Lanham, Md.: University Press of America, 1987), 117–29; and Albert R. Jonsen, "Casuistry as Methodology in Clinical Ethics," *Theoretical Medicine* 12 (1991): 295–307. I do not mean to imply, however, that the version of casuistic reasoning advocated by Jonsen and Toulmin is the same as the third approach discussed here.

28. Jonsen and Toulmin use the general term *circumstances* to refer to the morally relevant factors that can vary from case to case. I use the term *casuistic factors* in order to focus on those circumstances that are especially pertinent to resolving a type of case.

29. I have provided a detailed example of casuistic reasoning in "Justification in Ethics."

30. Kevin Wm. Wildes, "The Priesthood of Bioethics and the Return of Casuistry," *Journal of Medicine and Philosophy* 18 (1993): 33–49.

31. John D. Arras, "Getting Down to Cases: The Revival of Casuistry in Bioethics," *Journal of Medicine and Philosophy* 16 (1991): 29–51.

32. Ibid., 45–46.

33. Tom Tomlinson, "Casuistry in Medical Ethics: Rehabilitated, or Repeat Offender?" *Theoretical Medicine* 15 (1994): 5–20.

34. Strong, "Justification In Ethics," 195, 201–7.

35. Tomlinson, "Casuistry in Medical Ethics," 14.

Chapter 5

1. These are actual cases of my colleague Jay S. Schinfeld, M.D. These cases and the issue of artificial insemination for single women are discussed in Carson Strong and Jay S. Schinfeld, "The Single Woman and Artificial Insemination by Donor," *Journal of Reproductive Medicine* 29 (1984): 293–99.

2. I use the terms *artificial insemination by donor* and *donor insemination* interchangeably. However, the latter term currently seems to be preferred, presumably because the abbreviation of the former, AID, is too similar to AIDS. Accordingly, more often I shall use the latter term.

3. Daniel Wikler and Norma J. Wikler, "Turkey-baster Babies: The Demedicalization of Artificial Insemination," *Milbank Quarterly* 69 (1991): 5–40.

4. Ibid., 25–26.

5. See, e. g., Francie Hornstein, "Children by Donor Insemination: A New Choice for Lesbians" and Renate Duelli Klein, "Doing It Ourselves: Self Insemination," in Rita Arditti, Renate Duelli Klein, and Shelley Minden, eds., *Test-tube Women: What Future for Motherhood?* (London: Pandora, 1984), 373–81, 382–90.

6. I. M. Cosgrove, "AID for Lesbians" (letter), *British Medical Journal* 2 (1979): 495. Cosgrove argues that because of this possible harm, physicians should not carry out requests for DI by lesbians.

7. Mary Warnock, *A Question of Life: The Warnock Report on Human Fertilisation and Embryology* (Oxford: Blackwell, 1984), 11.

8. Ibid.

9. Ibid., 23. Similar objections to DI for single women are made by D. H. Wilson, "AID for Lesbians" (letter), *British Medical Journal* 2 (1979): 669; and Burton Z. Sokoloff, "Alternative Methods of Reproduction," *Clinical Pediatrics* 26 (1987): 11–17.

10. Elizabeth Herzog and Cecelia E. Sudia, "Fatherless Homes: A Review of Research," *Children* 15 (1968): 177–82. See also Herzog and Sudia, "Children in Fatherless Families" in B. Caldwell and H. Ricciuti, eds., *Review of Child Development Research,* vol. 3 (Chicago: University of Chicago Press, 1973), 141–232.

11. Clark E. Vincent, "Implications of Changes in Male-Female Role Expectations for Interpreting M-F Scores," *Journal of Marriage and the Family* 28 (1966): 196–99.

12. Ibid.

13. Richard Green, "Sexual Identity of Thirty-seven Children Raised by Homosexual or Transsexual Parents," *American Journal of Psychiatry* 135 (1978): 692–97. See also Richard Green et al., "Lesbian Mothers and Their Children: A Comparison with Solo Parent Heterosexual Mothers and Their Children," *Archives of Sexual Behavior* 15 (1986): 167–84.

14. Martha Kirkpatrick, Catherine Smith, and Ron Roy, "Lesbian Mothers and Their

Children: A Comparative Survey," *American Journal of Orthopsychiatry* 51 (1981): 545–51.

15. Beverly Hoeffer, "Children's Acquisition of Sex-role Behavior in Lesbian-mother Families," *American Journal of Orthopsychiatry* 51 (1981): 536–44; Susan Golombok, Ann Spencer, and Michael Rutter, "Children in Lesbian and Single-parent Households: Psychosexual and Psychiatric Appraisal," *Journal of Child Psychology and Psychiatry* 24 (1983): 551–72; Fiona Tasker and Susan Golombok, "Adults Raised as Children in Lesbian Families," *American Journal of Orthopsychiatry* 65 (1995): 203–15.

16. Lonnie G. Nungesser, "Theoretical Bases for Research on the Acquisition of Social Sex-roles by Children of Lesbian Mothers," *Journal of Homosexuality* 5 (1980): 177–87.

17. Ibid.

18. Karen Gail Lewis, "Children of Lesbians: Their Point of View," *Social Work* 25 (1980): 198–203.

19. Marcel Saghir and Eli Robins, *Male and Female Homosexuality* (Baltimore: Williams and Wilkins, 1973), 236.

20. Virginia O'Leary, "Lesbianism," *Nursing Dimensions* 7 (1979): 78–82; Serena Nanda and J. Scott Francher, "Culture and Homosexuality: A Comparison of Long-Term Gay Male and Lesbian Relationships," *Eastern Anthropologist* 33 (1980): 139–52.

21. R. A. Basile, "Lesbian Mothers," *Women's Rights Law Reporter* 2 (1974): 3–18; Sophie Freud Loewenstein, "Understanding Lesbian Women," *Social Casework* 61 (1980): 29–38.

22. Joel Feinberg, *Harm to Others* (New York: Oxford University Press, 1984), 31–64; and "Wrongful Life and the Counterfactual Element in Harming," *Social Philosophy and Policy* 4 (1987): 145–78.

23. Feinberg, "Wrongful Life," 149. Feinberg's discussion is much more extensive; this is only one of six conditions he specifies that are necessary and sufficient for harming. Also, Feinberg points out that a certain type of unusual situation is possible, referred to as causal overdetermination. The possibility of this type of situation requires a modification to the necessary condition in question, but that modification does not affect the analysis provided herein. See "Wrongful Life," 150–53.

24. Ibid., 158–59.

25. Fetal alcohol syndrome occurs in 30 to 40 percent of children born to women who are alcoholics. See F. Gary Cunningham et al., *Williams Obstetrics,* 19th ed. (Norwalk, Conn.: Appleton & Lange, 1993), 973–74.

26. Michael D. Bayles, "Harm to the Unconceived," *Philosophy and Public Affairs* 5 (1976): 292–304; Feinberg, *Harm to Others,* 99; Bonnie Steinbock and Ron McClamrock, "When Is Birth Unfair to the Child?" *Hastings Center Report* 24 (1994): 15–21.

27. Feinberg, "Wrongful Life," 168. The example is derived from Derek Parfit, "On Doing the Best for Our Children" in Michael D. Bayles, ed., *Ethics and Population* (Cambridge, Mass.: Schenkman, 1976), 100–115.

28. Feinberg, "Wrongful Life," 169.

29. Strong and Schinfeld, "Single Woman."

30. I do not mean to imply that there are important disadvantages, but rather that the task of justifying DI for single women is not as difficult as it often is believed to be.

31. Susan R. Johnson, Elaine M. Smith, and Susan M. Guenther, "Parenting Desires

among Bisexual Women and Lesbians," *Journal of Reproductive Medicine* 32 (1987): 198–200.

32. Edward M. Connor et al., "Reduction of Maternal-Infant Transmission of Human Immunodeficiency Virus Type 1 with Zidovudine Treatment," *New England Journal of Medicine* 331 (1994): 1173–80; The European Collaborative Study, "Caesarean Section and Risk of Vertical Transmission of HIV-1 Infection," *Lancet* 343 (1994): 1464–67; Cunningham et al., *Williams Obstetrics,* 1310–13.

33. Behniz Pakizegi, "Emerging Family Forms: Single Mothers by Choice—Demographic and Psychosocial Variables," *Maternal-Child Nursing Journal* 19 (1990): 1–19; Deborah I. Frank and Margaret H. Brackley, *Clinical Nurse Specialist* 3 (1989): 156–60.

34. See, e. g., Mark V. Sauer, Richard Paulson, and Rogerio A. Lobo, "Reversing the Natural Decline in Human Fertility: An Extended Clinical Trial of Oocyte Donation to Women of Advanced Reproductive Age," *Journal of the American Medical Association* 268 (1992): 1275–79.

35. "Italian Has Seven-pound Baby Boy at Age Sixty-two," Memphis *Commercial Appeal,* July 19, 1994: A2; Margaret Carlson, "Old Enough to Be Your Mother," *Time* 143 (Jan. 10, 1994): 41.

36. "I'll Be a Good Mother, Says Sixty-one-year-old," Memphis *Commercial Appeal,* Dec. 29, 1993: A4. Rossana Dalla Corte became the oldest birth mother on record since the time of the biblical story of Sarah, who was infertile. In that story, God made a covenant with Abraham, according to which he would be the ancestor of many nations. To fulfill the covenant, God enabled Abraham's wife, Sarah, to become pregnant at age ninety, and she gave birth to Isaac. *Genesis* 17: 1–24; 18: 1–15.

37. Carlson, "Old Enough," 41.

38. William Drozdiak, "France Seeks to Prohibit Retirement Pregnancies," Memphis *Commercial Appeal,* Jan. 4, 1994: A1, A9.

39. "Too Old at Fifty-nine?" *Nature* 367 (1994): 2; "Medical Advances Spur Debate over Reproductive Rights of Older Women," Memphis *Commercial Appeal,* Jan. 1, 1994: A1, A11.

40. This is not meant to be an exhaustive list, but it identifies some of the main complications addressed in the literature. See, e.g., Cunningham et al., *Williams Obstetrics,* 653–59; Gertrude S. Berkowitz et al., "Delayed Childbearing and the Outcome of Pregnancy," *New England Journal of Medicine* 322 (1990): 659–64; William N. Spellacy, Stephen J. Miller, and Ann Winegar, "Pregnancy after Forty Years of Age," *Obstetrics and Gynecology* 68 (1986): 452–54; Deborah K. Lehmann and James Chism, "Pregnancy Outcome in Medically Complicated and Uncomplicated Patients Aged Forty Years or Older," *American Journal of Obstetrics and Gynecology* 157 (1987): 738–42. *Placenta previa* refers to a placenta located in the lower part of the uterus, so that it partially or completely covers the cervical opening. Dilation of the cervix can then cause tearing of placental tissue and bleeding. Hemorrhage on the fetal side of the placenta can cause fetal death or brain damage as a result of asphyxia. When *placenta previa* is diagnosed during labor, cesarean section is necessary to save the fetus's life and minimize maternal bleeding. *Abruptio placentae* refers to premature separation of the placenta from the uterus. This condition also can lead to fetal blood loss with resulting brain damage or death. When *abruptio placentae* and fetal distress are diagnosed during labor, prompt cesarean delivery is necessary.

41. Mark V. Sauer, Richard J. Paulson, and Rogerio A. Lobo, "Pregnancy after Age Fifty: Application of Oocyte Donation to Women after Natural Menopause," *Lancet* 341 (1993): 321–23

42. For example, some U.S. Supreme Court justices have served in their eighties; some people have swum the English Channel in their sixties.

43. U.S. Bureau of the Census, *Statistical Abstract of the United States: 1992*, 112th ed. (Washington: Government Printing Office, 1992), 77. Life expectancies in other countries will differ from those in the United States.

44. We know that there are increased *genetic* risks to offspring of older women, such as an increased incidence of Down syndrome. These risks, however, are avoided when ova are donated by younger women.

45. See, e. g., *Griswold v. Connecticut* 381 U.S. 479; *Eisenstadt v. Baird* 405 U.S. 438; *Roe v. Wade* 410 U.S. 113; *Planned Parenthood of Southeastern Pennsylvania v. Casey* 120 L. Ed. 674.

46. *Skinner v. Oklahoma* 316 U.S. 535, 541.

47. *Loving v. Virginia* 388 U.S. 1.

48. *Stanley v. Illinois* 405 U.S. 645.

49. *Stanley v. Illinois* 405 U. S. 645, 651, citations deleted.

50. When IVF is unsuccessful for women over forty years of age, another approach is possible — IVF using ova donated by younger women.

51. *In the Matter of Baby M* 537 A.2d 1227 (N.J. 1988), 542 A.2d 52 (N.J. Super. Ch. 1988).

52. In commercial surrogacy, the infertile couple sometimes is referred to as the commissioning couple.

53. Arizona Revised Statutes Annotated, §25–218 (1989).

54. Congregation for the Doctrine of the Faith, "Instruction on Respect for Human Life in Its Origin and on the Dignity of Procreation," *Origins* 16 (1987): 697, 699–711. This document sets forth official views of the Roman Catholic church on procreation. Because of its lengthy title, the document is referred to as *Donum Vitae* after its first two Latin words.

55. Utah Code Annotated, §76–7–204 (1992 Cumulative Supplement).

56. The second view also has been advocated by several authors: George G. Annas, "Fairy Tales Surrogate Mothers Tell"; Alexander M. Capron and Margaret J. Radin, "Choosing Family Law over Contract Law as a Paradigm for Surrogate Motherhood"; and R. Alta Charo, "Legislative Approaches to Surrogate Motherhood" in Larry Gostin, ed., *Surrogate Motherhood: Politics and Privacy* (Bloomington: Indiana University Press, 1990), 43–55, 59–76, and 88–119.

57. New Hampshire Revised Statutes Annotated, chap. 168-B (1992 Cumulative Supplement).

58. For other expressions of the third view, see Ruth Macklin, "Is There Anything Wrong with Surrogate Motherhood? An Ethical Analysis," in Gostin, *Surrogate Motherhood*, 136–50; Code of Virginia, §§20–156, –165 (1992 Cumulative Supplement).

59. This Model Surrogacy Act is reprinted, in part, in Gostin, *Surrogate Motherhood*, Appendix 3, 270–80.

60. John A. Robertson, "Surrogate Mothers: Not So Novel After All," *Hastings Center Report* 13 (1983): 28–34; Bonnie Steinbock, "Surrogate Motherhood as Prenatal Adop-

tion," in Gostin, *Surrogate Motherhood,* 123–35; Lori B. Andrews, "Legal and Ethical Aspects of New Reproductive Technologies," *Clinical Obstetrics and Gynecology* 29 (1986): 190–204; Laura M. Purdy, "Surrogate Mothering: Exploitation or Empowerment?" *Bioethics* 3 (1989): 18–34.

61. *In the Matter of Baby M.*

62. *Johnson v. Calvert* 19 Cal. Rptr. 2d 494 (Cal. 1993).

63. Martha A. Field, *Surrogate Motherhood* (Cambridge, Mass.: Harvard University Press, 1988), 1–2.

64. See, e. g., Gena Corea, "Junk Liberty" in Gostin, *Surrogate Motherhood,* 325–37; and Susan Ince, "Inside the Surrogate Industry" in Arditti, Klein, and Minden, *Test-tube Women,* 99–116.

65. Lori B. Andrews, "Surrogate Motherhood; The Challenge for Feminists" in Gostin, *Surrogate Motherhood,* 167–82.

66. Elizabeth S. Anderson, "Is Women's Labor a Commodity?" *Philosophy and Public Affairs* 19 (1990): 71–92.

67. Debra Satz, "Markets in Women's Reproductive Labor," *Philosophy and Public Affairs* 21 (1992): 107–31.

68. Purdy, "Surrogate Mothering," 28.

69. Satz, "Markets," 125; Sara Ann Ketchum, "Selling Babies and Selling Bodies," *Hypatia* 4 (1989): 116–27; Susan Dodds and Karen Jones, "Surrogacy and Autonomy," *Bioethics* 3 (1989): 1–17.

70. Laura M. Purdy, "A Response to Dodds and Jones," *Bioethics* 3 (1989): 40–44.

71. Corea, "Junk Liberty."

Chapter 6

1. George P. Smith II, "Australia's Frozen Orphan Embryos: A Medical, Legal, and Ethical Dilemma," *Journal of Family Law* 24 (1985–86): 27–41.

2. *Davis v. Davis* 842 S.W. 2d 588 (Tenn. 1992).

3. National Institutes of Health, *Final Report of the Human Embryo Research Panel* (Bethesda, Md.: NIH, Sept. 27, 1994).

4. Associated Press, "Embryo Research Sparks Debate," *AP Online,* Sept. 28, 1994, V0442.

5. Louisiana Revised Statutes Annotated, Chap. 3, §§9:121–133.

6. C. R. Austin, *Human Embryos* (Oxford: Oxford University Press, 1989), 1–41; Clifford Grobstein, "The Early Development of Human Embryos," *Journal of Medicine and Philosophy* 10 (1985): 213–36.

7. Also, if two preembryos are combined at this stage, a single individual will develop. It will have genetic mosaicism, with cells consisting of two genetically different cell lines, derived from the two original preembryos. This fusing of preembryos has been accomplished experimentally in laboratory animals; see Ethics Committee of the American Fertility Society, "Ethical Considerations of the New Reproductive Technologies," *Fertility and Sterility* 53 (1990), suppl. 2, 31S.

8. The term *frozen embryo* often is used to refer to frozen preembryos. As discussed below, *frozen preembryo* is more accurate.

9. Attempts have been made to culture rat and mouse blastocysts in vitro beyond the

implantation stage, but development proceeds only for a short period and not in a normal manner; see Austin, *Human Embryos,* 36–38.

10. The distinction between potential to *cause* self-consciousness and potential to *become* self-conscious is discussed in Chap. 3.

11. Ethics Committee of the American Fertility Society, "Ethical Considerations of the New Reproductive Technologies," *Fertility and Sterility* 46 (1986), suppl. 1, 29S–30S. In 1995, the American Fertility Society changed its name to the American Society for Reproductive Medicine.

12. Congregation for the Doctrine of the Faith, "Instruction on Respect for Human Life in Its Origin and on the Dignity of Procreation," *Origins* 16 (1987): 701. Many of the objections to uses of preembryos discussed in this chapter are found in *Donum Vitae.*

13. Roger Wertheimer, "Understanding the Abortion Argument," *Philosophy and Public Affairs* 1 (1971): 82–83; Richard A. McCormick, "Who or What Is the Preembryo?" *Kennedy Institute of Ethics Journal* 1 (1991): 1–15.

14. Wertheimer, "Understanding the Abortion Argument," 76. It should be noted that in the history of Catholic writings there has been disagreement concerning when ensoulment, and hence personhood, begins. Thomas Aquinas argued that the soul is not present until animation, which is detected when the mother feels fetal movement (quickening). In his view, ensoulment and animation occur at 40 days gestational age for males and 80 days for females. This view was overturned by Pope Sixtus V, who declared that abortion at any time during gestation violates canon law. Later, Pope Gregory XIV repealed the penalties set forth by Sixtus V, except for abortions of an ensouled 40-day-old embryo. The history of Catholic doctrine is discussed in Harmon L. Smith, "Abortion — The Theological Tradition" in Robert L. Perkins, ed., *Abortion: Pro and Con* (Cambridge, Mass.: Schenkman, 1974), 37–51.

15. *York v. Jones* 717 F. Supp. 421 (E.D. Va. 1989). Also see Frank Feldinger, "Cryo-Babies in Court," *California Lawyer* 9 (August 1989): 19–20.

16. Rosemarie Tong, *Feminine and Feminist Ethics* (Belmont, Calif.: Wadsworth, 1993), 167–68.

17. Wendy Dullea Bowie, "Multiplication and Division — New Math for the Courts: New Reproductive Technologies Create Potential Legal Time Bombs," *Dickinson Law Review* 95 (1990): 155–81; Robert J. Muller, *"Davis v. Davis:* The Applicability of Privacy and Property Rights to the Disposition of Frozen Preembryos in Intrafamilial Disputes," *University of Toledo Law Review* 24 (1993): 763–804.

18. *York v. Jones,* 427.

19. Patricia A. Martin and Martin L. Lagod, "The Human Preembryo, the Progenitors, and the State: Toward a Dynamic Theory of Status, Rights, and Research Policy," *High Technology Law Journal* 5 (1990): 257–310, 270.

20. Freezing might also improve success rates by permitting transfer at a later cycle when superovulatory drugs are not being given. There is a possibility that such drugs reduce implantation rates; see Ethics Committee of the American Fertility Society, "Ethical Considerations of the New Reproductive Technologies," *Fertility and Sterility* 53, suppl. 2 (1990): 58S.

21. Congregation for the Doctrine of the Faith, "Instruction on Respect," 703.

22. Jacques Testart et al., "Factors Influencing the Success Rate of Human Embryo

Freezing in an In Vitro Fertilization and Embryo Transfer Program," *Fertility and Sterility* 48 (1987): 107–12; Jacques Cohen et al., "Cryopreservation of Zygotes and Early Cleaved Human Embryos," *Fertility and Sterility* 49 (1988): 283–89; Michel Camus et al., "Human Embryo Viability after Freezing with Dimethylsulfoxide as a Cryoprotectant," *Fertility and Sterility* 51 (1989): 460–65.

23. R. G. Edwards et al., "The Growth of Human Pre-implantation Embryos In Vitro," *American Journal of Obstetrics and Gynecology* 141 (1981): 408–16; Alexander Lopata, "Concepts in Human In Vitro Fertilization and Embryo Transfer," *Fertility and Sterility* 40 (1983): 289–301. There is evidence that preembryo viability is affected by several factors, including the method of superovulation and the presence of observable abnormal structures before freezing; see Testart et al., "Factors Influencing," 107–12; Cohen et al., "Cryopreservation," 283–89; and J. Mandelbaum et al., "Cryopreservation of Human Embryos and Oocytes," *Human Reproduction* 3 (1988): 117–19.

24. Congregation for the Doctrine of the Faith, Instruction on Respect, 704–5.

25. Other ethical arguments are given, but they include premises to the effect that it is God's judgment that certain actions are wrong. For example, so-called natural law arguments rest on the view that it is God's judgment that natural law should be obeyed.

26. Clifford Grobstein, Michael Fowler, and John Mendeloff, "Frozen Embryos: Policy Issues," *New England Journal of Medicine* 312 (1985): 1584–88.

27. Congregation for the Doctrine of the Faith, Instruction on Respect, 704–5.

28. Ibid., 705.

29. Ibid.

30. Jose Elizalde, "Bioethics as a New Human Rights Emphasis in European Research Policy," *Kennedy Institute of Ethics Journal* 2 (1992): 159–70, 161.

31. Peter Singer et al., eds., *Embryo Experimentation* (Cambridge: Cambridge University Press, 1990), Appendix 1, "A Summary of Legislation Relating to IVF," 227–45, 229; Louisiana Revised Statutes Annotated, Chapter 3, §9:122.

32. P. R. Braude, V. N. Bolton, and M. H. Johnson, "The Use of Human Pre-embryos for Infertility Research" in Gregory Bock and Maeve O'Connor, eds., *Human Embryo Research: Yes or No?* (London: Tavistock, 1986), 63–76.

33. Karen Dawson, "Introduction: An Outline of Scientific Aspects of Human Embryo Research" in Singer et al., *Embryo Experimentation*, 3–13, 9.

34. Testart et al., "Factors Influencing," 107–12; Cohen et al., "Cryopreservation," 283–89; Camus et al., "Human Embryo Viability," 460–65.

35. Alan Trounsen, "Why Do Research on Human Pre-embryos?" in Singer et al., *Embryo Experimentation*, 14–25, 15.

36. Braude, Bolton, and Johnson, "Use of Human Pre-embryos," 72–73.

37. R. J. Aitken and D. W. Lincoln, "Human Embryo Research: The Case for Contraception" in Bock and O'Connor, *Human Embryo Research*, 122–36.

38. Alan H. Handyside et al., "Birth of a Normal Girl after In Vitro Fertilization and Preimplantation Diagnostic Testing for Cystic Fibrosis," *New England Journal of Medicine* 327 (1992): 905–9.

39. Trounsen, "Why Do Research," 22.

40. Ibid., 22–23.

41. Robyn Rowland, "Making Women Visible in the Embryo Experimentation

Debate," *Bioethics* 1 (1987): 1–14; Robyn Rowland, *Living Laboratories: Women and Reproductive Technologies* (Bloomington: Indiana University Press, 1992).

42. See also Tong, *Feminine and Feminist Ethics,* 167–68.

43. See the essays in Patricia Spallone and Deborah Lynn Steinberg, eds., *Made to Order: The Myth of Reproductive and Genetic Progress* (Oxford: Pergamon, 1987). This is a collection of essays from a conference of FINRRAGE (Feminist International Network of Resistance to Reproductive and Genetic Engineering).

44. Gena Corea, "The Reproductive Brothel" in Gena Corea et al., eds., *Man-Made Women: How New Reproductive Technologies Affect Women* (London: Hutchinson, 1985), 38–51, 39.

45. National Institutes of Health, *Final Report of the Human Embryo Research Panel.*

46. Barbara Gregoratos, "Tempest in the Laboratory: Medical Research on Spare Embryos from *In Vitro* Fertilization," *Hastings Law Journal* 37 (1986): 977–1006; American Medical Association, Board of Trustees, "Frozen Pre-embryos," *Journal of the American Medical Association* 263 (1990): 2484–87.

47. This is similar to a recommendation in American College of Obstetricians and Gynecologists, Committee on Ethics, "Preembryo Research: History, Scientific Background, and Ethical Considerations," ACOG Committee Opinion Number 136, April 1994, 1–10.

48. Singer et al., *Embryo Experimentation,* 232–33, 238; Elizalde, "Bioethics as a New Human Rights Emphasis," 161; Louisiana Revised Statutes Annotated, Chapter 3, §9:122.

49. Dawson, Karen Dawson, "In Vitro Fertilisation: Legislation and Problems of Research," *British Medical Journal* 295 (1987).

50. Ibid., 1185.

51. See, e.g., United States Department of Health, Education and Welfare, Ethics Advisory Board, "HEW Support of Research Involving Human In Vitro Fertilization and Embryo Transfer," *Federal Register,* June 18, 1979: 35033–58; Victoria, Australia, Committee to Consider the Social, Ethical and Legal Issues Arising from In Vitro Fertilization, Louis Waller (chair), *Report on the Disposition of Embryos Produced by In Vitro Fertilization* (Melbourne: F. D. Atkinson Government Printer, 1984); Mary Warnock, *A Question of Life: The Warnock Report on Human Fertilisation and Embryology* (Oxford: Blackwell, 1984); LeRoy Walters, "Ethics and New Reproductive Technologies: An International Review of Committee Statements," *Hastings Center Report* 17 (June 1987): suppl., 3–9.

52. Alec Samuels, "Embryo Research: The Significance of the New Law," *Medicine, Science, and the Law* 31 (1991): 115–18.

53. Singer et al., *Embryo Experimentation,* 232.

54. Helga Kuhse and Peter Singer, "Individuals, Humans and Persons: The Issue of Moral Status" in Singer et al., *Embryo Experimentation,* 65–75; Peter Singer and Helga Kuhse, "The Ethics of Embryo Research," *Law, Medicine and Health Care* 14 (1986): 133–48.

55. K. J. S. Anand and P. R. Hickey, "Pain and Its Effects in the Human Neonate and Fetus," *New England Journal of Medicine* 317 (1987): 1321–29.

56. Singer and Kuhse suggest a 28-day limit in order to be very, very cautious in

avoiding research on sentient fetuses; see Singer and Kuhse, "Individuals," 74. However, given that the onset of sentience is very much later than 28 days, a 28-day limit has little plausible connection to sentience as a criterion.

57. Hans-Martin Sass, "Moral Dilemmas in Perinatal Medicine and the Quest for Large-Scale Embryo Research: A Discussion of Recent Guidelines in the Federal Republic of Germany," *Journal of Medicine and Philosophy* 12 (1987): 279–90, 285.

58. Ibid., 285.

59. As research in this area advances, it might some day be possible to maintain embryos in the laboratory beyond 14 days.

60. J. L. Hall et al., "Experimental Cloning of Human Polyploid Embryos Using an Artificial Zona Pellucida," *Fertility and Sterility* (1993), the American Fertility Society conjointly with the Canadian Fertility and Andrology Society, Program Supplement, S1.

61. Howard W. Jones, Jr., "Reflections on the Usefulness of Embryo Cloning," *Kennedy Institute of Ethics Journal* 4 (1994): 205–7.

62. Hall, "Experimental Cloning," S1.

63. Austin, *Human Embryos,* 45–48.

64. Rebecca Voelker, "A Clone by Any Other Name Is Still an Ethical Concern," *Journal of the American Medical Association* 271 (1994): 331–32.

65. Ibid., 332.

66. After publication of the results of their blastomere separation study in abstract form, it came to light that Hall and Stillman had not obtained approval for the study from the Institutional Review Board at their institution, George Washington University. Following an investigation of this breach of ethical rules, the university ordered the researchers to destroy their data. See Ruth Macklin, "Cloning without Prior Approval: A Response to Recent Disclosures of Noncompliance," *Kennedy Institute of Ethics Journal* 5 (1995): 57–60.

67. After fertilization, preembryos retain their totipotency only through the next two or three cell divisions. Somehow, a sort of cellular count takes place to keep track of this, and the count does not start over when blastomere separation occurs. It seems likely, therefore, that only about four viable preembryos can be obtained. Further separations can be performed but probably will not result in viable preembryos because the totipotency is lost. See Jacques Cohen and Giles Tomkin, "The Science, Fiction, and Reality of Embryo Cloning," *Kennedy Institute of Ethics Journal* 4 (1994): 193–203.

68. Karen Farkas, "Frozen Embryos Become Point of Dispute in Divorce," Cleveland *Plain Dealer,* Sept. 27, 1989: 1A, 22A.

69. American Medical Association, "Frozen Pre-embryos," 2487.

70. Duress is one of several recognized grounds for legally voiding a contract; see *Restatement of Contracts (Second),* § 367(1), 1979.

71. In the Davis case, Mary Sue later remarried and decided that she preferred to donate the preembryos to another infertile couple. If we apply our casuistic approach, we find that in this case it favors freedom not to procreate, given that Mary Sue had the option of attempting procreation with her new spouse. Thus, the casuistic approach supports carrying out Junior's request to discard the preembryos. This in fact was the decision reached by the Tennessee Supreme Court; see *Davis v. Davis* 842 S.W. 2d 588 (Tenn. 1992).

72. Warnock, *Question of Life,* 56.

73. P. H. Glenister and Mary F. Lyon, "Long-Term Storage of Eight-Cell Mouse Embryos at −196°C," *Journal of in Vitro Fertilization and Embryo Transfer* 3 (1986): 20–27.

74. The pros and cons of oocyte donation for older women were discussed in Chap. 5.

Chapter 7

1. Alan H. Handyside et al., "Birth of a Normal Girl after In Vitro Fertilization and Preimplantation Diagnostic Testing for Cystic Fibrosis," *New England Journal of Medicine* 327 (1992): 905–9; Gina Kolata, "Genetic Defects Detected in Embryos Just Days Old," *New York Times,* Sept. 24, 1992: A1. Preimplantation sex selection to avoid X-linked diseases also has been reported in Alan H. Handyside et al., "Pregnancies from Biopsied Human Preimplantation Embryos Sexed by Y-specific DNA Amplification," *Nature* 344 (1990): 768–70.

2. Yuet Wai Kan, "Development of DNA Analysis for Human Diseases: Sickle Cell Anemia and Thalassemia as a Paradigm," *Journal of the American Medical Association* 267 (1992): 1532–36.

3. Jane Gitshier et al., "Detection and Sequence of Mutations in the Factor VIII Gene of Haemophiliacs," *Nature* 315 (1985): 427–30.

4. M. Koenig et al., "Complete Cloning of the Duchenne Muscular Dystrophy (DMD) cDNA and Preliminary Genomic Organization of the DMD Gene in Normal and Affected Individuals," *Cell* 50 (1987): 509–17.

5. Margaret R. Wallace et al., "Type 1 Neurofibromatosis Gene: Identification of a Large Transcript Disrupted in Three NF1 Patients," *Science* 249 (1990): 181–86; David Viskochil et al., "Deletions and a Translocation Interrupt a Cloned Gene at the Neurofibromatosis Type 1 Locus," *Cell* 62 (1990): 187–92; Richard M. Cawthon et al., "A Major Segment of the Neurofibromatosis Type 1 Gene: cDNA Sequence, Genomic Structure, and Point Mutations," *Cell* 62 (1990): 193–201.

6. Huntington's Disease Collaborative Research Group, "A Novel Gene Containing a Trinucleotide Repeat That Is Expanded and Unstable on Huntington's Disease Chromosomes," *Cell* 72 (1993): 971–83.

7. John R. Riordan et al., "Identification of the Cystic Fibrosis Gene: Cloning and Characterization of Complementary DNA," *Science* 245 (1989): 1066–73.

8. European Polycystic Kidney Disease Consortium, "The Polycystic Kidney Disease 1 Gene Encodes a 14 kb Transcript and Lies within a Duplicated Region on Chromosome 16," *Cell* 77 (1994): 881–94.

9. Judy C. Chang and Yuet Wai Kan, "A Sensitive New Prenatal Test for Sickle-Cell Anemia," *New England Journal of Medicine* 307 (1982): 30–32; Wanda K. Lemna et al., "Mutation Analysis for Heterozygote Detection and the Prenatal Diagnosis of Cystic Fibrosis," *New England Journal of Medicine* 322 (1990): 291–96; Multicenter Study Group, "Diagnosis of Duchenne and Becker Muscular Dystrophies by Polymerase Chain Reaction: A Multicenter Study," *Journal of the American Medical Association* 267 (1992): 2609–15; Scott C. Kogan, Marie Doherty, and Jane Gitschier, "An Improved Method for Prenatal Diagnosis of Genetic Diseases by Analysis of Amplified DNA Sequences," *New England Journal of Medicine* 317 (1987): 985–90.

10. Petros Tsipouras et al., "Genetic Linkage of the Marfan Syndrome, Ectopia Lentis, and Congenital Contractural Arachnodactyly to the Fibrillin Genes on Chromosomes 15 and 5, *New England Journal of Medicine* 326 (1992): 905–9.

11. Departments of Health and Human Services and Energy, *Understanding Our Genetic Inheritance: The U.S. Human Genome Project: The First Five Years, FY 1991–1995* (Washington, D.C.: Government Printing Office, 1990), 1.

12. Eric T. Juengst, "The Human Genome Project and Bioethics," *Kennedy Institute of Ethics Journal* 1 (1991): 71–74.

13. Jeff M. Hall et al., "Linkage of Early-onset Familial Breast Cancer to Chromosome 17q21," *Science* 250 (1990): 1684–89; Yoshio Miki et al., "A Strong Candidate for the Breast and Ovarian Cancer Susceptibility Gene BRCA1,' *Science* 266 (1994): 66–71.

14. Joanna Groden et al., "Identification and Characterization of the Familial Adenomatous Polyposis Coli Gene," *Cell* 66 (1991): 589–600; Kenneth W. Kinzler et al., "Identification of FAP Locus Genes from Chromosome 5q21," *Science* 253 (1991): 661–5; Richard Fischel et al., "The Human Mutator Gene Homolog MSH2 and Its Association with Hereditary Nonpolyposis Colon Cancer," *Cell* 75 (1993): 1027–38.

15. Sotirios K. Karathanasis, Vassilis I. Zannis, and Jan L. Breslow, "A DNA Insertion in the Apolipoprotein A-I Gene of Patients with Premature Atherosclerosis," *Nature* 305 (1983): 823–25.

16. George S. Eisenbarth, "Type I Diabetes Mellitus: A Chronic Autoimmune Disease," *New England Journal of Medicine* 314 (1986): 1360–68.

17. Janice A. Egeland et al., "Bipolar Affective Disorders Linked to DNA Markers on Chromosome 11," *Nature* 325 (1987): 783–87.

18. Jill Murrell et al., "A Mutation in the Amyloid Precursor Protein Associated with Hereditary Alzheimer's Disease," *Science* 254 (1991): 97–99; R. Sherrington et al., "Cloning of a Gene Bearing Missense Mutations in Early-onset Familial Alzheimer's Disease," *Nature* 375 (1995): 754–60.

19. Francis S. Collins, "Medical and Ethical Consequences of the Human Genome Project," *Journal of Clinical Ethics* 2 (1991): 260–67.

20. Parts of this chapter are adapted from Carson Strong, "Tomorrow's Prenatal Genetic Testing: Should We Test for Minor Diseases?" *Archives of Family Medicine* 2 (1993): 1187–93; and Strong, "Genetic Screening in Oocyte Donation: Ethical and Legal Aspects" in Cynthia B. Cohen, ed., *New Ways of Making Babies: The Case of Egg Donation* (Bloomington, Ind.: Indiana University Press, 1996), 122–37.

21. There are, of course, other issues involving genetics in reproductive medicine. One of the first that received attention is the issue of when to introduce new tests into routine practice, and much of the discussion has focused on CF. An early consensus was reached that the mere availability of a CF test is not sufficient grounds for employing it in population or prenatal screening. Rather, additional conditions should first be met, including improvements in the predictive value of the test, assured quality control of laboratories conducting the test, and improved resources for educating and counseling those receiving the test. See, e.g., NIH Workshop on Population Screening for the Cystic Fibrosis Gene, "Special Report: Statement from the National Institutes of Health Workshop on Population Screening for the Cystic Fibrosis Gene," *New England Journal of Medicine* 323 (1990): 70–71. To explore how to bring about these conditions, the NIH has initiated a multidisciplinary three-year research project to define the best methods of educating and

counseling individuals who want to be tested for CF mutations. See Elinor J. Langfelder, Eric T. Juengst, and Elizabeth Thomson, "NIH Initiates Clinical Studies on Cystic Fibrosis Testing, Education, and Counseling," *Human Genome News,* January 1992: 1–2. This research is expected to culminate in a comprehensive report concerning the introduction of CF testing into practice. I shall not discuss this topic here because of space limitations and the fact that it already is receiving a great deal of attention from others.

22. President's Commission for the Study of Ethical Problems in Medicine and Biomedical and Behavioral Research, *Screening and Counseling for Genetic Conditions* (Washington, D.C.: Government Printing Office, 1983), 57–58; Eric T. Juengst, "Prenatal Diagnosis and the Ethics of Uncertainty" in John F. Monagle and David C. Thomasma, eds., *Medical Ethics: A Guide for Health Professionals* (Rockville, Md.: Aspen, 1988), 12–25.

23. Ruth R. Faden et al., "Prenatal Screening and Pregnant Women's Attitudes toward the Abortion of Defective Fetuses," *American Journal of Public Health* 77 (1987): 288–90; Mark I. Evans et al., "Attitudes on the Ethics of Abortion, Sex Selection, and Selective Pregnancy Termination among Health Care Professionals, Ethicists, and Clergy Likely to Encounter Such Situations," *American Journal of Obstetrics and Gynecology* 164 (1991): 1092–99.

24. Collins, "Medical and Ethical Consequences," 266.

25. Ibid., 266; Geoffrey Cowley, "Made to Order Babies," *Newsweek* 114, special issue (Winter 1990): 94–100.

26. If amniocentesis were used, fetal cells usually would be obtained at sixteen to nineteen weeks' gestational age. If chorionic villus sampling (CVS), early amniocentesis, or fetal cell sorting were used, the cells would be obtained even earlier in pregnancy. If we assume that two weeks would be needed to analyze the cells following amniocentesis and that less time would be needed following CVS, then most abortions would occur earlier than twenty weeks' gestational age. Moreover, data on the neurological development of the fetus suggests that sentience could not be present prior to approximately twenty to twenty-four weeks' gestational age. See K. J. S. Anand and P. R. Hickey, "Pain and Its Effects in the Human Neonate and Fetus," *New England Journal of Medicine* 317 (1987): 1321–29.

27. Angus Clarke, "Is Non-directive Genetic Counselling Possible?" *Lancet* 338 (1991): 998–1001.

28. Stephen G. Post, Jeffrey R. Botkin, and Peter Whitehouse, "Selective Abortion for Familial Alzheimer Disease?" *Obstetrics and Gynecology* 79 (1992): 794–8. For a similar view, see American Medical Association Council on Ethical and Judicial Affairs, "Ethical Issues Related to Prenatal Genetic Testing," *Archives of Family Medicine* 3 (1994): 633–42.

29. W. French Anderson, "Human Gene Therapy: Why Draw a Line?" *Journal of Medicine and Philosophy* 14 (1989): 681–93.

30. President's Commission, *Screening and Counseling,* 55.

31. Ibid., 37; Juengst, "Prenatal Diagnosis," 19.

32. Daniel J. Kevles, *In the Name of Eugenics: Genetics and the Uses of Human Heredity* (New York: Knopf, 1985).

33. Albert Edward Wiggam, *The Fruit of the Family Tree* (Indianapolis: Bobbs-Merrill, 1925).

34. Elyce Zenoff Ferster, "Eliminating the Unfit — Is Sterilization the Answer?" *Ohio State Law Journal* 27 (1966): 591–633.

35. Robert N. Proctor, *Racial Hygiene: Medicine under the Nazis* (Cambridge, Mass.: Harvard University Press, 1988).

36. Ferster, "Eliminating the Unfit," 632.

37. Mark W. Steele and W. Roy Breg, Jr., "Chromosome Analysis of Human Amniotic-Fluid Cells," *Lancet* 1 (1966): 383–85.

38. President's Commission, *Screening and Counseling,* 38; Clarke, "Is Non-directive Genetic Counselling Possible?" 998–1001.

39. Louis J. Elsas II, "A Clinical Approach to Legal and Ethical Problems in Human Genetics," *Emory Law Journal* 39 (1990): 811–53.

40. See, e.g., Dorothy C. Wertz and John C. Fletcher, "Sex Selection in India," *Hastings Center Report* 19 (1989): 25.

41. Diana W. Bianchi et al., "Isolation of Fetal DNA from Nucleated Erythrocytes in Maternal Blood," *Proceedings of the National Academy of Sciences* 87 (1990): 3279–83; Sherman Elias et al., "First Trimester Prenatal Diagnosis of Trisomy 21 in Fetal Cells from Maternal Blood," *Lancet* 340 (1992): 1033.

42. Jeffrey R. Botkin, "Prenatal Screening: Professional Standards and the Limits of Parental Choice," *Obstetrics and Gynecology* 75 (1990): 875–80.

43. A similar argument in the context of germ line genetic modification can be found in Burke K. Zimmerman, "Human Germ-Line Therapy: The Case for Its Development and Use," *Journal of Medicine and Philosophy* 16 (1991): 593–612.

44. Concerns about positive eugenics are expressed in the following: Anderson, "Human Gene Therapy," 681–93; Dorothy C. Wertz and John C. Fletcher, "Fatal Knowledge? Prenatal Diagnosis and Sex Selection," *Hastings Center Report* 19 (1989): 21–27; "A Report from Germany: An Extract from Prospects and Risks of Gene Technology: The Report of the Enquete Commission to the Bundestag of the Federal Republic of Germany," *Bioethics* 2 (1988): 254–63.

45. Ronald Munson and Lawrence H. Davis, "Germ-line Gene Therapy and the Medical Imperative," *Kennedy Institute of Ethics Journal* 2 (1992): 137–58.

46. "Report from Germany," 260.

47. *Berman v. Allan* 404 A.2d 8 (N.J. 1979).

48. *Roe v. Wade* 410 U.S. 113 (1973).

49. Martin M. Quigley, Robert L. Collins, and Leslie R. Schover, "Establishment of an Oocyte Donor Program: Donor Selection and Screening," *Annals of the New York Academy of Sciences* 626 (1991): 445–51; Mark V. Sauer and Richard J. Paulson, "Human Oocyte and Preembryo Donation: An Evolving Method for the Treatment of Infertility," *American Journal of Obstetrics and Gynecology* 163 (1990): 1421–24; Christine Kilgore, "Egg Donation Programs Facing Ethical Issues, Donor Shortage: Potential for Ovum Banks," *Ob. Gyn. News,* Feb. 1–14, 1990: 1, 14.

50. Amitai Etzioni, "Sex Control, Science, and Society," *Science* 161 (1968): 1107–12.

51. Michael Bayles, *Reproductive Ethics* (Englewood Cliffs, N.J.: Prentice-Hall, 1984), 35.

52. Wertz and Fletcher, "Fatal Knowledge?" 24.

53. Mary Anne Warren, *Gendercide* (Totowa, N.J.: Rowman and Allanheld, 1985), 83–88.

54. Martin Curie-Cohen, Lesleigh Luttrell, and Sander Shapiro, "Current Practice of Artificial Insemination by Donor in the United States," *New England Journal of Medicine* 300 (1979): 585–90.

55. William G. Johnson, Robin C. Schwartz, and Abe M. Chutorian, "Artificial Insemination by Donors: The Need for Genetic Screening," *New England Journal of Medicine* 304 (1981): 755–77.

56. M. Chrystie Timmons et al., "Genetic Screening of Donors for Artificial Insemination," *Fertility and Sterility* 35 (1981): 451–56.

57. F. Clarke Fraser and R. Allan Forse, "On Genetic Screening of Donors in Artificial Insemination," *American Journal of Medical Genetics* 10 (1981): 399–405.

58. See, e.g., Joe Leigh Simpson, "Genetic Screening for Donors in Artificial Insemination by Donor," *Fertility and Sterility* 35 (1981): 395–96; Marion S. Verp, Melvin R. Cohen, and Joe Leigh Simpson, "Necessity of Formal Genetic Screening in Artificial Insemination by Donor," *Obstetrics and Gynecology* 62 (1983): 474–79; J. Selva et al., "Genetic Screening for Artificial Insemination by Donor (AID)," *Clinical Genetics* 29 (1986) 389–96; Ethics Committee of the American Fertility Society, "Ethical Considerations" (1986), 36S–44S, 83S–84S; Ethics Committee of the American Fertility Society, "Ethical Considerations" (1990), 43S–50S, 88S–89S.

59. American Fertility Society, "Guidelines for Gamete Donation: 1993," *Fertility and Sterility* 59 (1993), suppl 1.: 1S–9S.

60. Although there is considerable agreement among the various sets of guidelines that have been put forward, also there are differences. For example, Timmons and colleagues recommend that if two or more stillbirths, fetal deaths, or unexplained neonatal deaths occur in a first-degree relative, then further investigation should be performed to rule out a genetic cause; however, neither Fraser and Forse nor the AFS guidelines include this recommendation. Also, Selva and colleagues recommend routine karyotyping of donors, but Fraser and Forse claim that it is not warranted. It is worth noting that the various authors and committees do not point out how their guidelines differ from previously published ones, nor do they defend their version over others. For example, Verp and coworkers do not explain why they chose not to include Fraser and Forse's recommendation that a donor be rejected if there is a first-degree relative with a chromosomal abnormality, unless the donor is known to have a normal karyotype. Thus, within this literature there has been little critical assessment of opposing views.

61. Common familial diseases are covered by the guidelines referring to major multifactorial, polygenic, and autosomal dominant disorders.

62. Natalie Angier, "Scientists Isolate Novel Gene Linked to Colon Cancer," *New York Times*, Dec. 3, 1993: A1.

63. Ibid.

64. Ibid.

65. Ethics Committee of the American Fertility Society, "Ethical Considerations" (1986); Ethics Committee of the American Fertility Society, "Ethical Considerations" (1990).

66. U.S. Congress, Office of Technology Assessment, *Artificial Insemination: Practice in the United States: Summary of a 1987 Survey — Background Paper* (Washington, D.C.: Government Printing Office, 1988), 40–41, 64–65, 67, 72–73.

67. Ibid., 67.

68. See, e.g., Susan C. Klock and Donald Maier, "Psychological Factors Related to Donor Insemination," *Fertility and Sterility* 56 (1991): 489–95; and Leslie R. Schover, Robert L. Collins, and Susan Richards, "Psychological Aspects of Donor Insemination: Evaluation and Follow-up of Recipient Couples," *Fertility and Sterility* 57 (1992): 583–90.

69. U.S. Congress, Office of Technology Assessment, *Artifical Insemination,* 41.

70. Ibid., 72–73.

71. Quigley, Collins, and Schover, "Establishment of an Oocyte Donor Program," 447.

72. Andrea Mechanic Braverman, "Survey Results on the Current Practice of Ovum Donation," *Fertility and Sterility* 59 (1993): 1216–20.

73. Kilgore, "Egg Donation Programs," 1, 14.

Chapter 8

1. *Roe v. Wade* 410 U.S. 113 (1973).

2. The term *tocolytic* means labor-arresting. Fetal monitoring involves measurement of the fetal heart rate. Certain patterns of fetal heart rate in relation to uterine contractions, as well as very low heart rate, are considered evidence of fetal hypoxia, which can result in fetal death or brain damage. Such heart-rate patterns are regarded as medical indications for cesarean section.

3. This case is discussed in Terrence F. Ackerman and Carson Strong, *A Casebook of Medical Ethics* (New York: Oxford University Press, 1989), 71–75. Parts of this chapter are adapted from Carson Strong, "Ethical Conflicts between Mother and Fetus in Obstetrics," *Clinics in Perinatology* 14 (1987): 313–28; Carson Strong, "Delivering Hydrocephalic Fetuses," *Bioethics* 5 (1991); Carson Strong, "An Ethical Framework for Managing Fetal Anomalies in the Third Trimester," *Clinical Obstetrics and Gynecology* 35 (1992): 792–802; and Carson Strong and Garland D. Anderson, "An Ethical Framework for Issues during Pregnancy" in Raanan Gillon, ed., *Principles of Health Care Ethics* (Chichester: Wiley, 1994), 587–600.

4. Under the heading "beneficent actions," I include actions that prevent, remove, or avoid causing harm, as well as actions that positively benefit others. See William K. Frankena, *Ethics,* 2d ed. (Englewood Cliffs, N.J.: Prentice-Hall, 1973), 45–48.

5. The term *innocent* is used because killing seems to be justifiable in certain situations such as self-defense against an attacker or in a just war, but these examples involve killing persons who have given up their innocence by their own actions.

6. See, e. g., Willard Gaylin et al, "Doctors Must Not Kill," *Journal of the American Medical Association* 259 (1988): 2139–40.

7. For some authors, the principle of avoiding killing falls under the more general principle of nonmaleficence, which in turn is regarded by some as coming under the principle of beneficence. However, the principle of avoiding killing should be identified explicitly and considered separately from the principle of beneficence, for several reasons. First, the moral significance of killing is not reducible to considerations of beneficence. For example, killing destroys not only the well-being of persons but also their autonomy. Second, killing can have legal ramifications that have great practical significance to

decisions by the physician. Explicit discussion of killing draws our attention to these legal considerations.

8. In support of this claim, it seems plausible to say that we have obligations to certain individuals to act beneficently toward them, even though they are not persons in the normative sense. For example, to inflict pain unnecessarily on animals is cruel and wrong. However, it also is plausible to say that our obligations toward normative persons are stronger. For example, there are research studies in which it is ethically justifiable to expose laboratory animals, but not humans, to risk of harm.

9. Part of what it means to say that an individual has a diminished moral standing compared to persons in the normative sense is that its right to life (if it has such a right) is less strong than that of persons in the normative sense. A possible objection is that consequentialist considerations might support a very strong duty to avoid killing a fetus, even though it has a diminished moral standing. However, it should be remembered that my argument for conferred moral standing is based on consequentialist considerations. A diminished moral standing is justified precisely because a diminished similarity with the paradigm implies that the consequentialist argument for avoiding killing is less strong than it is for individuals who are highly similar to the paradigm.

10. Paul Benjamin Linton, "Enforcement of State Abortion Statutes after *Roe*: A State-by-state Analysis," *University of Detroit Law Review* 67 (1990): 157–259.

11. Ibid.; David Manchester et al., "Management of Pregnancies with Suspected Fetal Anomalies: Clinical Experience and Ethical Issues" in Carl Nimrod and Glenn Griener, eds., *Biomedical Ethics and Fetal Therapy* (Waterloo, Ont.: Wilfred Laurier University Press, 1988), 67–79.

12. Linton, "Enforcement of State Abortion Statutes," passim.

13. It might be objected that if abortion is not locally available or seems beyond the means of a particular patient, then the physician need not mention it as an option. In reply, a patient might be helped in thinking through her decision by knowing about the limited availability of abortion. Moreover, some patients might have resources, such as a source of borrowed funds, of which the physician is unaware. Respect for autonomy suggests that it is better to disclose than to withhold this information.

14. See, e. g., Michael R. Harrison et al., "Successful Repair In Utero of a Fetal Diaphragmatic Hernia after Removal of Herniated Viscera from the Left Thorax," *New England Journal of Medicine* 322 (1990): 1582–84; Kim M. Davidson et al., "Successful In Utero Treatment of Fetal Goiter and Hypothyroidism," *New England Journal of Medicine* 324 (1991): 543–46; and Richard P. Porreco et al., "Palliative Fetal Surgery for Diaphragmatic Hernia," *American Journal of Obstetrics and Gynecology* 170 (1994): 833–34.

15. In the future, it is possible that advances in fetal therapy will alter this state of affairs, making fetal therapy before viability more common.

16. *Roe v. Wade* 410 U.S. 113, 160 (1973).

17. *Roe v. Wade*, 163.

18. *Colautti v. Franklin* 439 U.S. 379, 58 L. ed. 2d 596, 604 (1979).

19. *Planned Parenthood of Missouri v. Danforth* 428 U.S. 52, 49 L. ed. 788, 802 (1976).

20. *Colautti v. Franklin*, 605.

21. Carson Strong, "Ethical Framework for Managing Fetal Anomalies," 797.

22. Joyce L. Peabody, Janet R. Emery, and Stephen Ashwal, "Experience with Anencephalic Infants as Prospective Organ Donors," *New England Journal of Medicine* 321 (1989): 344–50.

23. Gary McAbee et al., "Prolonged Survival of Two Anencephalic Infants," *American Journal of Perinatology* 10 (1993): 175–77.

24. George J. Annas, "Asking the Courts to Set the Standard of Emergency Care — The Case of Baby K," *New England Journal of Medicine* 330 (1994): 1542–45.

25. F. Gary Cunningham et al., *Williams Obstetrics,* 19th ed. (Norwalk, Conn.: Appleton & Lange, 1993), 920.

26. Kenneth Lyons Jones, ed., *Smith's Recognizable Patterns of Human Malformation* (Philadelphia: Saunders, 1988), 17, 20. See also R. Redheendran, R. L. Neu, and R. M. Bannerman, "Long Survival in Trisomy-13-Syndrome: 21 Cases Including Prolonged Survival in Two Patients 11 and 19 Years Old," *American Journal of Medical Genetics* 8 (1981): 167–72; and C. F. Geiser and A. M. Schindler, "Long Survival in a Male with 18-Trisomy Syndrome and Wilms Tumor," *Pediatrics* 44 (1969): 111–16.

27. This discussion constitutes an argument against the view of McCullough and Chervenak. They claim that in the third trimester there are anomalies, including anencephaly, in which the physician should recommend that the pregnant woman choose either abortion or nonaggressive management. The legal considerations I have discussed provide reasons not to follow their approach of recommending abortion as an option in the third trimester in cases involving anencephaly. See, e. g., Laurence B. McCullough and Frank A. Chervenak, *Ethics in Obstetrics and Gynecology* (New York: Oxford University Press, 1994),211–23; Frank A. Chervenak and Laurence B. McCullough, "An Ethically Justified, Clinically Comprehensive Management Strategy for Third-Trimester Pregnancies Complicated by Fetal Anomalies," *Obstetrics and Gynecology* 75 (1990): 311–16.

28. Cunningham et al., *Williams Obstetrics,* 514. See also J. H. Edwards, "Congenital Malformations of the Nervous System in Scotland," *British Journal of Preventive and Social Medicine* 12 (1958): 115–30; and Rustin McIntosh et al., "The Incidence of Congenital Malformations: A Study of 5,964 Pregnancies," *Pediatrics* 14 (1954): 505–21.

29. David C. McCullough and Lynn A. Balzer-Martin, "Current Prognosis in Overt Neonatal Hydrocephalus," *Journal of Neurosurgery* 57 (1982): 378–83; John Mealey, Jr., Richard L. Gilmor, and Michael P. Bubb, "The Prognosis of Hydrocephalus Overt at Birth," *Journal of Neurosurgery* 39 (1973): 348–55; R. O. Weller and Kenneth Shulman, "Infantile Hydrocephalus: Clinical, Histological, and Ultrastructural Study of Brain Damage," *Journal of Neurosurgery* 36 (1972): 255–65; R. C. Rubin et al., "The Effect of Severe Hydrocephalus on Size and Number of Brain Cells," *Developmental Medicine and Child Neurology* 14, suppl. 27 (1972): 117–20.

30. Cunningham et al., *Williams Obstetrics,* 514; K. H. Nicolaides et al., "Fetal Lateral Cerebral Ventriculomegaly: Associated Malformations and Chromosomal Defects," *Fetal Diagnosis and Therapy* 5 (1990): 5–14; Arie Drugan et al., "The Natural History of Prenatally Diagnosed Cerebral Ventriculomegaly," *Journal of the American Medical Association* 261 (1989): 1785–88; Roger J. Hudgins et al., "Natural History of Fetal Ventriculomegaly," *Pediatrics* 82 (1988): 692–97; Anthony M. Vintzileos et al., "Perinatal

Management and Outcome of Fetal Ventriculomegaly," *Obstetrics and Gynecology* 69 (1987): 5–11; David A. Nyberg et al., "Fetal Hydrocephalus: Sonographic Detection and Clinical Significance of Associated Anomalies," *Radiology* 163 (1987): 187–91; Frank A. Chervenak et al., "The Management of Fetal Hydrocephalus," *American Journal of Obstetrics and Gynecology* 151 (1985): 933–41; Michael R. Harrison, Mitchell S. Golbus, and Roy A. Filly, *The Unborn Patient* (Orlando: Grune and Stratton, 1984), 349–77; Roger A. Williamson et al., "Heterogeneity of Prenatal Onset Hydrocephalus: Management and Counseling Implications," *American Journal of Medical Genetics* 17 (1984): 497–508.

31. Harrison, Golbus, and Filly, *Unborn Patient,* 363.

32. Charles M. McCurdy, Jr., and John W. Seeds, "Route of Delivery of Infants with Congenital Anomalies," *Clinics in Perinatology* 20 (1993): 81–106; William H. Clewell et al., "Ventriculomegaly: Evaluation and Management," *Seminars in Perinatology* 9 (1985): 98–102.

33. John R. Evrard and Edwin M. Gold, "Cesarean Section and Maternal Mortality in Rhode Island," *Obstetrics and Gynecology* 50 (1977): 594–97; George L. Rubin et al., "Maternal Death after Cesarean Section in Georgia," *American Journal of Obstetrics and Gynecology* 139 (1981): 681–85; Diana B. Petitti et al., "In-Hospital Maternal Mortality in the United States: Time Trends and Relation to Method of Delivery," *Obstetrics and Gynecology* 59 (1982): 6–12; Benjamin P. Sachs et al., "Cesarean Section–Related Maternal Mortality in Massachusetts, 1954–1985," *Obstetrics and Gynecolocy* 71 (1988): 385–88; R. J. Lilford, "The Relative Risks of Caesarean Section (Intrapartum and Elective) and Vaginal Delivery: A Detailed Analysis to Exclude the Effects of Medical Disorders and Other Acute Pre-existing Physiological Disturbances," *British Journal of Obstetrics and Gynaecology* 97 (1990): 883–92.

34. Watson A. Bowes, Jr., et al., "Breech Delivery: Evaluation of the Method of Delivery on Perinatal Results and Maternal Morbidity," *American Journal of Obstetrics and Gynecology* 135 (1979): 965–73. See also Joseph M. Miller, Jr., "Maternal and Neonatal Morbidity and Mortality in Cesarean Section," *Obstetrics and Gynecology Clinics of North America* 15:4 (1988): 629–38; and Robert E. Rogers, "Complications of Cesarean Section," *Obstetrics and Gynecology Clinics of North America* 15:4 (1988): 673–84.

35. Thorkild F. Nielsen and Klas-Henry Hökegård, "Cesarean Section and Intraoperative Surgical Complications," *Acta Obstetrica et Gynecologica Scandinavica* 63 (1984): 103–8.

36. Chervenak et al., "Management of Fetal Hydrocephalus"; Frank A. Chervenak and Roberto Romero, "Is There a Role for Fetal Cephalocentesis in Modern Obstetrics?" *American Journal of Perinatology* 1 (1984): 170–73; Donald J. McCrann and Barry S. Schifrin, "Heart Rate Patterns of the Hydrocephalic Fetus," *American Journal of Obstetrics and Gynecology* 117 (1973): 69–74; David D. Cochrane and S. Terence Myles, "Management of Intrauterine Hydrocephalus," *Journal of Neurosurgery* 57 (1982): 590–96.

37. Chervenak and Romero, "Is There a Role for Fetal Cephalocentesis?"

38. McCrann and Schifrin, "Heart Rate Patterns." A late deceleration is a type of drop in fetal heart rate following a uterine contraction. Beat-to-beat variability is the normal

variation in instantaneous fetal heart rate. Late decelerations and loss of beat-to-beat variability indicate fetal asphyxia.

39. M. Amato et al., "Fetal Ventriculomegaly Due to Isolated Brain Malformations," *Neuropediatrics* 21 (1990): 130–32; Drugan et al., "Natural History"; Hudgins et al., "Natural History of Fetal Ventriculomegaly"; Vintzileos et al., "Perinatal Management"; Willy Serlo et al., "Prognostic Signs in Fetal Hydrocephalus," *Child's Nervous System* 2 (1986): 93–97; Chervenak et al., "Management of Fetal Hydrocephalus"; Dolores H. Pretorius et al., "Clinical Course of Fetal Hydrocephalus: 40 Cases," *AJR* (American Journal of Roentgenology) 144 (1985): 827–31.

40. I discuss several of these studies in Carson Strong, "Defective Infants and Their Impact on Families: Ethical and Legal Considerations," *Law, Medicine, and Health Care* 2 (1983): 168–72, 181.

41. Harrison, Golbus, and Filly, *Unborn Patient,* 363, 371.

42. Ibid., 349, 366.

43. I discuss the issue of coercive treatment when the pregnant woman refuses cesarean section for fetal hydrocephaly in Carson Strong, "Maternal Rights, Fetal Harms," *Hastings Center Report* 21 (1991): 21–22.

44. Thanatophoric dysplasia is a lethal condition in which bones do not grow properly. It is characterized by marked shortening of limb bones. Cloverleaf skull refers to a distinctive three-lobed deformity in the top of the skull. Thanatophoric dysplasia can be diagnosed with a high degree of reliability when ultrasound examinations reveal extreme limb shortening and cloverleaf skull in a fetus whose parents have normal stature. See Barry S. Mahoney, "The Extremities" in David A. Nyberg, Barry S. Mahoney, and Dolores H. Pretorius, eds., *Diagnostic Ultrasound of Fetal Anomalies: Text and Atlas* (Chicago: Year Book Medical Publishers, 1990), 492–562, 506–7. In only two rare cases has survival beyond a short period been reported, in Ian M. MacDonald et al., "Growth and Development in Thanatophoric Dysplasia," *American Journal of Medical Genetics* 33 (1989): 508–12

45. Trisomy 13 and 18 syndromes can be diagnosed with high reliability by means of chromosome analysis. Alobar holoprosencephaly is a condition in which the cerebrum is made up of a single sphere rather than two hemispheres. It usually results in death soon after birth, but sometimes there is survival with profound cognitive deficit. When characteristic cranial and facial features are detected by ultrasound, the diagnosis can be made with a high degree of reliability. See Michael F. Greene, Beryl R. Benacerraf, and Fredric D. Frigoletto, Jr., "Reliable Criteria for the Prenatal Sonographic Diagnosis of Alobar Holoprosencephaly," *American Journal of Obstetrics and Gynecology* 156 (1987): 687–89.

46. The Dandy-Walker syndrome is a brain malformation characterized by a cyst-like enlargement of the fourth ventricle and complete or partial absence of the cerebellar vermis. Some infants survive and some do not, depending in part on the presence of other anomalies. See Paul D. Russ, Dolores H. Pretorius, and Mark J. Johnson, "Dandy-Walker Syndrome: A Review of Fifteen Cases Evaluated by Prenatal Sonography," *American Journal of Obstetrics and Gynecology* 161 (1989): 401–6. The current lack of reliability in diagnosing renal agenesis (absence of kidneys) is indicated in Roberto Romero et al.,

"Antenatal Diagnosis of Renal Anomalies with Ultrasound: III. Bilateral Renal Agenesis," *American Journal of Obstetrics and Gynecology* 151 (1985): 38–43.

47. Cunningham et al., *Williams Obstetrics,* 1166.

48. Ibid., 863.

49. F. Gary Cunningham, Paul C. MacDonald, and Norman F. Gant, eds., *Williams Obstetrics,* 18th ed. (Norwalk, Conn.: Appleton and Lange, 1989), 445.

50. R. D. Wilson, D. Hitchman, and B. K. Wittman, "Clinical Follow-up of Prenatally Diagnosed Isolated Ventriculomegaly, Microcephaly, and Encephalocele," *Fetal Therapy* 4 (1989): 49–57; Frank A. Chervenak et al., "Diagnosis and Management of Fetal Cephalocele," *Obstetrics and Gynecology* 64 (1984): 86–91.

51. Isao Date et al., "Long-Term Outcome in Surgically Treated Encephalocele," *Surgical Neurology* 40 (1993): 125–30; Philippe Jeanty et al., "Prenatal Diagnosis of Fetal Cephalocele: A Sonographic Spectrum," *American Journal of Perinatology* 8 (1991): 144–49; Indrajeet Kaur and Jagdishwari Mishra, "Occipital Encephalocele," *Journal of the Indian Medical Association* 83 (1985): 126–27; Donald A. Simpson, David J. David, and Julian White, "Cephaloceles: Treatment, Outcome, and Antenatal Diagnosis," *Neurosurgery* 15 (1984): 14–21; Chervenak et al., "Diagnosis and Management of Fetal Cephalocele"; Philip Weinstein et al., "Prenatal Diagnosis of Occipital Encephalocele by Ultrasound Scanning," *Neurosurgery* 12 (1983): 680–83; D. W. K. Man and D. M. Forrest, "The Prognosis of Occipital Encephalocele: Experience of 46 Cases," *Zeitschrift für Kinderchirurgie* 37 (1982): 158–60; John Lorber and Julia K. Schofield, "The Prognosis of Occipital Encephalocele," *Zeitschrift für Kinderchirurgie* 28 (1979): 347–51; A. N. Guthkelch, "Occipital Cranium Bifidum," *Archives of Disease in Childhood* 45 (1970): 104–9; John Mealey, Jr., Andrievs J. Dzenitis, and Arthur A. Hockey, "The Prognosis of Encephaloceles," *Journal of Neurosurgery* 32 (1970): 209–18; R. Lipschitz, J. M. Beck, and C. Froman, "An Assessment of the Treatment of Encephalomeningoceles," *South African Medical Journal* 43 (1969): 609–10.

52. Lorber and Schofield, "Prognosis of Occipital Encephalocele"; Mealey, Dzenitis, and Hockey, "Prognosis of Encephaloceles." Microcephaly is abnormal smallness of the head.

53. Simpson, David, and White, "Cephaloceles"; Guthkelch, "Occipital Cranium Bifidum."

54. Wilson, Hitchman, and Wittman, "Clinical Follow-up"; Chervenak et al., "Diagnosis and Management of Fetal Cephalocele."

55. Some authors have recommended routine cesarean section when the defect is small and there are no other serious anomalies, to avoid trauma to the neural tissue associated with vaginal delivery. See Charles M. McCurdy, Jr., and John W. Seeds, "Route of Delivery of Infants with Congenital Anomalies," *Clinics in Perinatology* 20:1 (1993): 81–106.

56. In repositioning, the woman is placed on her left side to relieve compression of the superior vena cava by the uterus, in an attempt to increase blood flow. Repositioning and oxygenation are routine noninvasive steps to try to remove fetal distress. Other cases in which it is reasonable for the physician to try to persuade the woman to accept a balancing approach after she has requested aggressive treatment in the face of lethal anomalies are discussed by Joseph A. Spinnato et al., "Aggressive Intrapartum Management

of Lethal Fetal Anomalies: Beyond Fetal Beneficence," *Obstetrics and Gynecology* 85 (1995): 89–92.

57. The Medical Task Force on Anencephaly, "The Infant with Anencephaly," *New England Journal of Medicine* 322 (1990): 669–74; P. A. Baird and A. D. Sadovnick, "Survival in Infants with Anencephaly," *Clinical Pediatrics* 23 (1984): 268–71.

58. Medical Task Force on Anencephaly, "Infant with Anencephaly."

Chapter 9

1. Watson A. Bowes, Jr., and Brad Selgestad, "Fetal versus Maternal Rights: Medical and Legal Perspectives," *Obstetrics and Gynecology* 58 (1981): 209–14.

2. For an explanation of the terms *late deceleration, beat-to-beat variability*, and *repositioning*, see Chap. 8, nn. 38 and 56. Asphyxia causes relaxation of the sphincter and release of meconium, the fetal bowel contents, into the amniotic fluid.

3. Placental abruption is a premature separation of the placenta from the uterus, and it is accompanied by bleeding. In *chronic* abruption, the bleeding stops before delivery, but there is a risk of further bleeding episodes. The amniotic membranes provide a barrier against microorganisms from the vagina; rupture of the membranes removes this barrier, and with passage of time there is an increasing risk of infection of the membranes and the in utero fetus.

4. This case is discussed in Carson Strong and Garland D. Anderson, "An Ethical Framework for Issues during Pregnancy" in Raanan Gillon, ed., *Principles of Health Care Ethics* (Chichester: Wiley, 1994). Parts of this chapter are adapted from that article and from Strong, "Court-ordered Treatment in Obstetrics: The Ethical Views and Legal Framework," *Obstetrics and Gynecology* 78 (1991): 861–68; and Strong, "Ethical Conflicts between Mother and Fetus in Obstetrics," *Clinics in Perinatology* 14 (1987): 313–28.

5. See, e. g., Bowes and Selgestad, "Fetal versus Maternal Rights"; Veronika E. B. Kolder, Janet Gallagher, and Michael T. Parsons, "Court-ordered Obstetrical Interventions," *New England Journal of Medicine* 316 (1987): 1192–96; *Jefferson v. Griffin Spalding County Hospital Authority*, 247 Ga. 86, 274 S.E. 2d 457 (1981); *In re Madyun* (Docket No. 189–86), D.C. Sup. Ct. Civ. Div., 25 June 1986, published as an appendix to Judge Belson's dissenting opinion at 573 A. 2d 1259; Frank A. Chervenak, Laurence B. McCullough, and Daniel W. Skupski, "An Ethical Justification for Emergency, Coerced Cesarean Delivery," *Obstetrics and Gynecology* 82 (1993): 1029–35.

6. *Application of Jamaica Hospital* 128 Misc. 2d 1006, 491 N.Y.S. 2d 898 (N.Y. Sup. Ct. 1985); Kolder, Gallagher, and Parsons, "Court-ordered Obstetrical Interventions."

7. Wendy Chavkin, "Mandatory Treatment for Drug Use during Pregnancy," *Journal of the American Medical Association* 266 (1991): 1556–61.

8. See, e. g., Wendy Chavkin and Stephen Kandall, "Between a Rock and a Hard Place: Perinatal Drug Abuse," *Pediatrics* 85 (1990): 223–25; Sandra Anderson Garcia, "Birth Penalty: Societal Response to Perinatal Chemical Dependence," *Journal of Clinical Ethics* 1 (1990): 135–40; and Kary Moss, "Substance Abuse during Pregnancy," *Harvard Women's Law Journal* 13 (1990): 278–99. Jennifer Johnson was also sentenced to 15 years of probation and 200 hours of community service.

9. Kolder, Gallagher, and Parsons, "Court-ordered Obstetrical Interventions."

10. *In re A. C.* 573 A. 2d 1235 (D.C. App. 1990). The precedent established in this case will be discussed below.

11. Kolder, Gallagher, and Parsons, "Court-ordered Obstetrical Interventions."

12. In that case, doctors at Chicago's St. Joseph Hospital recommended cesarean section because they believed that the placenta was not carrying enough oxygen to the fetus. The pregnant woman, Tabita Bricci, refused cesarean delivery, based on personal religious beliefs and her desire to carry the fetus to term. The juvenile court and the Illinois Appellate Court refused to order a cesarean section. See, e. g., "State Can't Force Woman to Have Caesarean Section, Illinois Appeals Panel Says," *Washington Post,* Dec. 15, 1993: A3.

13. See, e. g., Nancy K. Rhoden, "Cesareans and Samaritans," *Law, Medicine and Health Care* 15 (1987): 118–25; Dawn Johnsen, "A New Threat to Pregnant Women's Autonomy," *Hastings Center Report* 17 (1987): 33–40; Martha A. Field, "Controlling the Woman to Protect the Fetus," *Law, Medicine and Health Care* 17 (1989): 114–29; Laura M. Purdy, "Are Pregnant Women Fetal Containers?" *Bioethics* 4 (1990): 273–91; Janet Gallagher, "Prenatal Invasions and Interventions: What's Wrong with Fetal Rights?" *Harvard Women's Law Journal* 10 (1987): 9–58; Judith Kahn, "Of Woman's First Disobedience: Forsaking a Duty of Care to Her Fetus—Is This a Mother's Crime? *Brooklyn Law Review* 53 (1987): 807–43; Mary Anne Warren, "The Moral Significance of Birth," *Hypatia* 4 (1989): 46–65; Kolder, Gallagher, and Parsons, "Court-ordered Obstetrical Interventions"; Mary Mahowald, "Beyond Abortion: Refusal of Caesarean Section," *Bioethics* 3 (1980): 106–21; and Susan Goldberg, "Medical Choices during Pregnancy: Whose Decision Is It Anyway?" *Rutgers Law Review* 41 (1989): 591–623.

14. *Application of Jamaica Hospital,* 491 N.Y.S. 2d 898 (N.Y. Sup. Ct. 1985). Esophageal varices are enlarged esophageal veins that are superficial, thin-walled, and liable to massive hemorrhage.

15. Actually, the court record did not discuss these aspects of the *Jamaica* case.

16. *Taft v. Taft* 388 Mass. 331, 446 N.E. 2d 395 (1983).

17. *Jefferson v. Griffin Spalding County Hospital Authority,* 274 S.E. 2d 457 (1981); *Raleigh Fitkin–Paul Morgan Memorial Hospital v. Anderson* 42 N.J. 421, 201 A. 2d 537, *cert. denied* 377 U.S. 985 (1964).

18. George J. Annas, "Forced Cesareans: The Most Unkindest Cut of All," *Hastings Center Report* 12 (1982): 16–17, 45.

19. Gallagher, "Prenatal Invasions and Interventions."

20. Annas, "Forced Cesareans."

21. Ronna Jurow and Richard H. Paul, "Cesarean Delivery for Fetal Distress without Maternal Consent," *Obstetrics and Gynecology* 63 (1984): 596–98.

22. *In re A. C.,* 573 A. 2d 1235 (D.C. App 1990).

23. *In re A. C.,* 1237, emphasis added. I referred to this statement as legal dictum in an earlier article, "Court-ordered Treatment in Obstetrics: The Ethical Views and Legal Framework," pp. 863–64. However, I have reconsidered and no longer believe that it should be regarded as mere dictum. Rather, it is integral to the court's decision in *In re A. C.,* being part of the main legal framework set forth by the court in deciding the case. Thus, the claim that it should be regarded as a precedent is more strongly supported than I indicated in the earlier article.

24. *In re A. C.,* 1252, citations deleted.

25. See, e. g., William J. Curran, "Court-ordered Cesarean Sections Receive Judicial Defeat," *New England Journal of Medicine* 323 (1990): 489–92; George J. Annas, "Foreclosing the Use of Force: A. C. Reversed," *Hastings Center Report* 20 (1990): 27–29; Claire C. Obade, *"In Re A. C.* Reversed: Judicial Recognition of the Rights of Pregnant Women," *Journal of Clinical Ethics* 1 (1990): 251; Linda J. Gobbis, "Recent Developments in Health Law Relevant to Health Care Providers," *Nurse Practitioner* 17 (1992): 77–78, 80; and Gerard S. Letterie, Glenn R. Markenson, and Maria M. Markenson, "Discharge against Medical Advice in an Obstetric Unit," *Journal of Reproductive Medicine* 38 (1993): 370–74.

26. In discussing my article "Court-ordered Treatment in Obstetrics: The Ethical Views and Legal Framework," *Obstetrics and Gynecology* 78 (1991): 861–67, and my letter of the same title in *Obstetrics and Gynecology* 79 (1992): 478–79, Laurence B. McCullough and Frank A. Chervenak claimed that my discussion of *In re A. C.* contained several errors which undermined my conclusion that the case set a precedent giving strong weight to maternal autonomy in cases of maternal-fetal conflict. See McCullough and Chervenak, *Ethics in Obstetrics and Gynecology* (New York: Oxford University Press, 1994), 264, n. 39. Their claims do not defeat my conclusion, but it is necessary to respond to each of them because my discussion of *In re A. C.* in the earlier article is similar to my discussion of it in this chapter.

First, they claimed that I ignored legal scholarship that takes opposing views, notably John Robertson's work. Presumably, they were referring to Robertson's argument that if the pregnant woman chooses to continue her pregnancy beyond the point of viability, then she incurs a legal obligation to promote the well-being of the fetus. See, e. g., Robertson, "The Right to Procreate and In Utero Fetal Therapy," *Journal of Legal Medicine* 3 (1982): 333–66; "Legal Issues in Prenatal Therapy," *Clinical Obstetrics and Gynecology* 29 (1986): 603–11; and "Reconciling Offspring and Maternal Interests during Pregnancy" in Sherrill Cohen and Nadine Taub, eds., *Reproductive Laws for the 1990s* (Clifton, N.J.: Humana, 1989), 259–74. However, this argument does not defeat my claim that *In re A. C.* set the precedent in question, for several reasons. First, as I pointed out near the beginning of this chapter, the fact that the woman has an obligation to the fetus does not settle the question of whether forced interventions are justifiable. McCullough and Chervenak assume that it does, but to assume this without giving an argument is unwarranted. Second, although McCullough and Chervenak seem to make this unwarranted assumption, Robertson does not. In a more recent essay, which I cited in the earlier article, (p. 868, n. 32), he stated repeatedly that forced interventions during pregnancy would be justifiable only rarely, even though he continued to hold that the pregnant woman has an obligation to avoid harming the fetus. See John A. Robertson and Joseph D. Schulman, "Pregnancy and Prenatal Harm: The Case of Mothers with PKU," *Hastings Center Report* 13 (1987): 23–33. Thus, Robertson's position on this point does not constitute an objection to the view I defended.

Second, McCullough and Chervenak claim that I ignored the arguments given in *In re Madyun* (Docket No. 189–86), D.C. Sup. Ct. Civ. Div., 25 June 1986. But *Madyun* is a trial court, not an appellate court, decision. As such, its statements cannot constitute precedent in appellate court decisions. Although it was affirmed by the District of

Columbia Court of Appeals in an unpublished order, such affirmation does not confer precedential value upon a trial court decision. As stated in *American Jurisprudence*, "A decision of a reviewing court affirming the decision of a lower court, without an opinion on the legal point involved, cannot have stare decisis effect" (20 Am. Jur. 2d, Courts § 189, citation deleted).

Third, they assert that I distorted *In re A. C.* by ignoring the court's claim that no maternal-fetal conflict existed in that case and then applying its ruling to maternal-fetal conflicts. However, they erred in stating that the court claimed that there was no maternal-fetal conflict. It is possible that they misinterpreted the following statement by the court: "Thus there was no clear maternal-fetal conflict in this case arising from a competent decision by the mother to forego a procedure for the benefit of the fetus" (573 A. 2d 1235, 1243). Here the court is not claiming that there was no maternal-fetal conflict but is pointing out that because the competency of the patient was uncertain, there was no conflict *arising from a competent decision by the mother*. Later the court explicitly stated that the case of A. C. involved maternal-fetal conflict: "In this case . . . the medical interests of the mother and the fetus were in sharp conflict: what was good for one would have been harmful to the other" (p. 1252, n. 23).

Fourth, they claim that I distorted *In re A. C.* by omitting discussion of a dissenting opinion in which Judge Belson expressed reservations about the court's ruling and claimed that more weight should be given to the state's interest in protecting a viable fetus. In response, precedent is established by the majority opinion, not by a dissenting opinion. A dissenting opinion only constitutes legal dictum. Judge Belson's comments do not diminish the fact that a strong precedent was set by the majority to the effect that great weight should be given to maternal interests in maternal-fetal conflicts.

Fifth, they claim I distorted *In re A. C.* by stating that its ruling would be important for future cases. They believe that the view that it will be important is speculative and is undermined by the neutrality of the court in *In re A. C.* to *Madyun*, a dimension of *In re A. C.* that they claim I ignored. In reply, the decision in *In re A. C.* clearly will be important for future cases because it will have to be taken into account in discussions of precedent. The neutrality of the court in *In re A. C.* to *Madyun* consisted of its refraining from discussing whether *Madyun* was rightly or wrongly decided. This reflects nothing more than the propensity of courts to discuss only the issues necessary to resolve the case at hand. In the passages in which the court said that it would not comment on *Madyun*, it stated, "We see no need to reach out and decide an issue that is not presented on the record before us" (p. 1252). In fact, it seems that the court only mentioned *Madyun* because it was discussed in the dissenting opinion by Judge Belson. The court's refraining from discussing *Madyun* in no way undermines the precedent it set, and the fact that I did not discuss the court's neutrality concerning *Madyun* does not detract from my conclusions.

27. *Thornburgh v. American College of Obstetricians and Gynecologists* 476 U.S. 747, 90 L. ed. 2d 779 (1986).

28. Kolder, Gallagher, and Parsons, "Court-ordered Obstetrical Interventions"; Lawrence J. Nelson and Nancy Milliken, "Compelled Medical Treatment of Pregnant Women," *Journal of the American Medical Association* 259 (1988): 1060–66; Lawrence J. Nelson, Brian P. Buggy, and Carol J. Weil, "Forced Medical Treatment of Pregnant

Women: Compelling Each to Live as Seems Good to the Rest," *Hastings Law Journal* 37 (1986): 703–63; Nancy K. Rhoden, "The Judge in the Delivery Room," *California Law Review* 74 (1986): 1951–2030; Gallagher, "Prenatal Invasions and Interventions"; Janet Gallagher, "Fetus as Patient" in Sherrill Cohen and Nadine Taub, eds., *Reproductive Laws for the 1990s* (Clifton, N.J.: Humana, 1989), 185–235; Alice M. Noble-Algire, "Court-ordered Cesarean Sections: A Judicial Standard for Resolving the Conflict between Fetal Interests and Maternal Rights," *Journal of Legal Medicine* 10 (1989): 211–49; Goldberg, "Medical Choices during Pregnancy."

29. *Roe v. Wade* 410 U. S. 113 (1973).

30. *Thornburgh* 90 L. ed. 2d 779, 785.

31. *Thornburgh* 90 L. ed. 2d 779, 799; *American College of Obstetricians and Gynecologists v. Thornburgh* 737 F. 2d 283 (1984), 300.

32. Nelson and Milliken, "Compelled Medical Treatment of Pregnant Women"; Nelson, Buggy, and Weil, "Forced Medical Treatment of Pregnant Women"; Rhoden, "Judge in the Delivery Room"; Rhoden, "Cesareans and Samaritans"; Gallagher, "Prenatal Invasions and Interventions"; Gallagher, "Fetus as Patient." A more recent Supreme Court decision, *Planned Parenthood v. Casey,* 120 L. ed. 2d 674 (1992), opened the door to a possible challenge to this argument based on *Thornburgh.* In *Thornburgh,* the Court used a standard requiring strict scrutiny of all proposed restrictions on the right to abortion. In *Casey,* the Court rejected strict scrutiny of all restrictions in favor of a new undue burden standard. According to this standard, restrictions are unconstitutional if their purpose or effect is to place a substantial obstacle in the path of a woman seeking an abortion before the fetus attains viability (120 L. ed. 2d 674, 715). In the future, the Supreme Court might be asked to consider whether increased risks for the pregnant woman in the context of postviability abortion constitute an undue burden. Although it can be argued that the answer should be yes, it is not a certainty that this would be the Court's answer. However, in the absence of a Supreme Court decision that such risks are not an undue burden, the ruling in *Thornburgh* that it is unconstitutional to force a woman to undergo such risks remains law, and the argument based on *Thornburgh* is valid.

33. *Cruzan v. Director, Missouri Department of Health* 110 S. Ct. 2841, 111 L. ed. 2d 224 (1990).

34. *Roe v. Wade* 410 U. S. 113 (1973); *Cruzan v. Director, Missouri Department of Health* 111 L. ed. 2d 224 (1990); *Griswold v. Connecticut* 381 U. S. 479 (1965); *In re Quinlan* 70 N.J. 10, 355 A. 2d 647 (1976); *In re Conroy* 98 N.J. 321, 486 A. 2d 1209 (1985); *Conservatorship of Drabick* 200 Cal. App. 3d 185, 245 Cal. Rptr. 840 (1988).

35. In commenting on my earlier article "Court-ordered Treatment in Obstetrics," McCullough and Chervenak have claimed that I made several errors in relying on the argument based on *Thornburgh* (*Ethics in Obstetrics and Gynecology,* pp. 264–65, n. 39). Although none of their claims has merit, it is necessary to respond to each of them because my previous discussion of the argument based on *Thornburgh* is similar to that presented in this chapter.

First, McCullough and Chervenak claimed that I provided no argument to show that abortion cases are analogous to maternal-fetal conflicts. This claim ignores my discussion on p. 864, in which I argued for the analogy in question. Specifically, I raised and responded to an objection that the suggested legal analogy between situations involving abortion and those involving refusal of therapy does not hold.

Second, they claimed that the language of the Court in Cruzan is far from unequivocal in supporting a constitutionally protected right to refuse medical treatment. This claim by McCullough and Chervenak is an inaccurate description of the *Cruzan* decision. In its majority opinion, written by Chief Justice Rehnquist, the Court stated, "The principle that a competent person has a constitutionally protected liberty interest in refusing unwanted medical treatment may be inferred from our prior decisions" (111 L. ed. 2d 224, 241), and it then discussed briefly several prior decisions supporting this conclusion. On p. 242 the Court stated, "Still other cases support the recognition of a general liberty interest in refusing medical treatment," and the Court identified those Supreme Court cases. The Court went on to state, "But for purposes of this case, we assume that the United States Constitution would grant a competent person a constitutionally protected right to refuse lifesaving hydration and nutrition" (p. 242) and then, "It cannot be disputed that the Due Process Clause protects an interest in life as well as an interest in refusing life-sustaining medical treatment" (p. 243). Justice Scalia was the only one of nine justices to disagree with the proposition that there is a constitutionally protected right to refuse medical treatment. In separate opinions, Justices O'Connor and Stevens each explicitly endorsed the view that there is such a right, and Justices Brennan, Marshall, and Blackmun forcefully set forth arguments supporting that right. Although Justices Brennan, Marshall, and Blackmun characterized the Court's assertion of this right as tentative, presumably because the Court at one point said that it would *assume* that there is such a right, later they explained this statement by the Court. By assuming, for purposes of this case only, that a competent person has a constitutionally protected liberty interest in being free of unwanted artificial nutrition and hydration, the Court was avoiding discussing the extent and limits of the right to refuse medical treatment (pp. 257–58). Thus, the Court's use of the term *assume* should not be interpreted as indecisiveness by the majority over the question of whether there is a constitutionally protected right to refuse medical treatment. Taking into account these considerations, the view that the Court was far from unequivocal on the point in question represents an unsupportable reading of the case.

Third, they pointed out that Judge Belson stated the view, in a dissenting opinion in *In re A. C.,* p. 1258, n. 12, that it is unclear whether *Thornburgh* applies in cases of cesarean delivery at term. To respond, it is necessary to consider the rest of Judge Belson's comment, which consisted of a reference to Noble-Allgire, "Court-ordered Cesarean Sections," p. 239, where Noble-Allgire argued as follows: "Furthermore, even if the Supreme Court maintains its no trade off mandate for abortion cases such as *Thornburgh,* it can be argued that the rule should not be applied in the Cesarean delivery cases. One distinguishing factor is that in the abortion context, a woman is exercising her right to terminate the pregnancy and thus the courts need not give great consideration to the fetus [sic] health, but in the Cesarean section situation, the woman has chosen to have her child and should be required to undergo a surgical delivery if necessary for the fetus." A reply can be given to this argument, and hence to Judge Belson's comment. In stating that the courts need not give great consideration to the fetus's health, Noble-Allgire apparently is assuming that in post-viability pregnancy terminations to prevent serious maternal harm, the fetuses always die. However, one should not make this assumption. Depending on the gestational age, such terminations can result in a live-born infant. Such procedures are perhaps more accurately described as early deliveries rather than abortions. Thus, preserving the fetus's health can be a legitimate concern. Moreover, although Noble-Allgire stated that in the cesarean section cases the woman has chosen to have her child, presumably because she has continued the pregnancy past the point of viability, the same can be said concerning early deliveries to prevent serious maternal harm. The pregnant woman has chosen to have her child, given that she has carried the pregnancy beyond viability. When the fetus is relatively advanced in gestation, the pregnant woman in this type of situation often prefers a method of delivery that maximizes the chances of infant survival. In *Thornburgh*, the Court ruled that the *state* cannot *force* the pregnant woman to undergo increased risks in order to maximize the probability of fetal survival. These situations are similar to refusal-of-treatment cases in several legally relevant ways: both involve viable fetuses, conflicts between fetal well-being and maternal well-being and autonomy, and the use of state power to force the woman to bear increased risks for the sake of the fetus. These similarities are sufficient to suggest a legal analogy, and Noble-Allgire does not show that there are dissimilarities great enough to refute the argument based on *Thornburgh*.

Fourth, McCullough and Chervenak claimed that I ignored my own insistence that there is a strong prohibition against killing at-term fetuses and did not show how this squares with the application of *Thornburgh* to maternal-fetal conflicts. Apparently, they believe that fetal death resulting from maternal refusal of treatment would constitute killing, although it is not clear that it would. Even if it would, the application of *Thornburgh* to maternal-fetal conflicts does not absolutely preclude coerced interventions aimed at preventing fetal death. However, I have argued that although respect for fetal life near term is important, the burden of justifying such interventions is heavy.

36. Frank A. Chervenak and Laurence B. McCullough, "Clinical Guides to Preventing Ethical Conflicts between Pregnant Women and Their Physicians," *American Journal of Obstetrics and Gynecology* 162 (1990): 303–7.

37. See, e. g., E. Earlene Dal Pozzo and Frank H. Marsh, "Psychosis and Pregnancy: Some New Ethical and Legal Dilemmas for the Physician," *American Journal of Obstetrics and Gynecology* 156 (1987): 425–27; Thomas E. Elkins et al., "Court-ordered Cesarean Section: An Analysis of Ethical Concerns in Compelling Cases," *American Journal of Obstetrics and Gynecology* 161 (1989): 150–54; and *In re Steven S.* 126 Cal. App. 3d 23, 178 Cal. Rptr. 525 (1981).

38. Rhoden, "Judge in the Delivery Room"; Rhoden, "Cesareans and Samaritans."

39. "Some Forced Cesareans Called Justifiable," *Ob. Gyn. News* 24 (Nov. 15–30, 1989): 3, 30; Elkins et al., "Court-ordered Cesarean Section"; Frank A. Chervenak and Laurence B. McCullough, "Justified Limits on Refusing Intervention," *Hastings Center Report* 21 (1991): 12–18. In *complete,* or total, placenta previa, the internal cervical os is completely covered by placenta.

40. See, e. g., Nelson, Buggy, and Weil, "Forced Medical Treatment of Pregnant Women"; John C. Fletcher, "Drawing Moral Lines in Fetal Therapy," *Clinical Obstetrics and Gynecology* 29 (1986): 595–602; and M. L. Poland, Reproductive Technology and Responsibility, *International Journal of Moral and Social Studies* 1 (1986): 63–76.

41. Rhoden, "Judge in the Delivery Room," 1959.

42. In referring to my view, Chervenak, McCullough, and Skupski state that my criteria are so abstractly stated that they have no reliable clinical applicability ("Ethical Justification," 1030). However, it is simply inaccurate to characterize a casuistic approach as abstract. One of the strengths of casuistic reasoning is that it is based on actual cases rather than abstract principles. Also, the claim that my view lacks clinical applicability is mistaken. As I point out in the text below, my view provides a practical rule of thumb for obstetricians: Don't override the competent obstetric patient's autonomy. This gives the correct answer in almost every case, and thus it has high clinical applicability. However, a rule of thumb is not necessarily absolute, and clinicians must use their judgment in identifying the truly exceptional case. The fact that this might sometimes be difficult does not make it abstract. Casuistry makes no pretense to resolve all hard cases.

43. Ira J. Chasnoff, "Drug Use and Women: Establishing a Standard of Care," *Annals of the New York Academy of Sciences* 562 (1989): 208–10; Mark G. Neerhof et al., "Cocaine Abuse during Pregnancy: Peripartum Prevalence and Perinatal Outcome," *American Journal of Obstetrics and Gynecology* 161 (1989): 633–38; Ira J. Chasnoff, Harvey J. Landress, and Mark E. Barrett, "The Prevalence of Illicit-drug or Alcohol Use during Pregnancy and Discrepancies in Mandatory Reporting in Pinellas County, Florida," *New England Journal of Medicine* 322 (1990): 1202–6; Deborah A. Frank et al., "Cocaine Use during Pregnancy: Prevalence and Correlates," *Pediatrics* 82 (1988): 888–95; Sherry K. George et al., "Drug Abuse Screening of Childbearing-age Women in Alabama Public Health Clinics," *American Journal of Obstetrics and Gynecology* 165 (1991): 924–27; Patrick Reddin, Barbara Schlimmer, and Connie Mitchell, "Cocaine and Pregnant Women: A Hospital Study," *Iowa Medicine* 81 (1991): 374–76; Enrique M. Ostrea, Jr., et al., "Drug Screening of Newborns by Meconium Analysis: A Large-Scale, Prospective, Epidemiologic Study," *Pediatrics* 89 (1992): 107–13.

44. American Medical Association Board of Trustees, "Legal Interventions during Pregnancy: Court-ordered Medical Treatments and Legal Penalties for Potentially Harmful Behavior by Pregnant Women," *Journal of the American Medical Association* 264 (1990): 2663–70; Arden Handler et al., "Cocaine Use during Pregnancy: Perinatal Outcomes," *American Journal of Epidemiology* 133 (1991): 818–25; Ira J. Chasnoff et al., "Cocaine Use in Pregnancy," *New England Journal of Medicine* 313 (1985): 666–69; Mitchell P. Dombrowski et al., "Cocaine Abuse Is Associated with Abruptio Placentae and Decreased Birth Weight, But Not Shorter Labor," *Obstetrics and Gynecology* 77 (1991): 139–41; H. R. Cohen, J. R. Green, and W. R. Crombleholme, "Peripartum Cocaine Use: Estimating Risk of Adverse Pregnancy Outcome," *International Journal of Gynecology and Obstetrics* 35 (1991): 51–54.

45. American Medical Association Board of Trustees, "Legal Interventions during Pregnancy"; Scott N. MacGregor et al., "Cocaine Use during Pregnancy: Adverse Perinatal Outcomes," *American Journal of Obstetrics and Gynecology* 157 (1987): 686–90; Amy S. Oro and Suzanne D. Dixon, "Perinatal Cocaine and Methamphetamine Exposure: Maternal and Neonatal Correlates," *Journal of Pediatrics* 111 (1987): 571–78; Michelle Chouteau, Pearila Brickner Namerow, and Phyllis Leppert, "The Effect of Cocaine Abuse on Birth Weight and Gestational Age," *Obstetrics and Gynecology* 72 (1988): 351–54; Bertis B. Little et al., "Cocaine Abuse during Pregnancy: Maternal and

Fetal Implications," *Obstetrics and Gynecology* 73 (1989): 157–60; Ira J. Chasnoff et al., "Temporal Patterns of Cocaine Use in Pregnancy: Perinatal Outcome," *Journal of the American Medical Association* 261 (1989): 1741–44; Arthur T. Evans and Kathy Gillogley, "Drug Use in Pregnancy: Obstetric Perspectives," *Clinics in Perinatology* 18 (1991): 23–32; Anthony J. Hadeed and Sharon R. Siegel, "Maternal Cocaine Use during Pregnancy: Effect on the Newborn Infant," *Pediatrics* 84 (1989): 205–10; Nesrin Bingol et al., "Teratogenicity of Cocaine in Humans," *Journal of Pediatrics* 110 (1987): 93–96; Stephen E. Lipshultz, Joseph J. Frassica, and E. John Orav, "Cardiovascular Abnormalities in Infants Prenatally Exposed to Cocaine," *Journal of Pediatrics* 118 (1991): 44–51; Gilberto F. Chávez, Joseph Mulinare, and José F. Cordero, "Maternal Cocaine Use during Early Pregnancy as a Risk Factor for Congenital Urogenital Anomalies," *Journal of the American Medical Association* 262 (1989): 795–98; Cohen, Green, and Crombleholme, "Peripartum Cocaine Use"; Richard R. Viscarello et al., "Limb-body Wall Complex Associated with Cocaine Abuse: Further Evidence of Cocaine's Teratogenicity," *Obstetrics and Gynecology* 80 (1992): 523–26.

46. Tatiana M. Doberczak et al., "Neonatal Neurologic and Electroencephalographic Effects of Intrauterine Cocaine Exposure," *Journal of Pediatrics* 113 (1988): 354–58; Suzanne D. Dixon, "Effects of Transplacental Exposure to Cocaine and Methamphetamine on the Neonate," *Western Journal of Medicine* 150 (1989): 436–42; Cathy Strachan Lindenberg et al., "A Review of the Literature on Cocaine Abuse in Pregnancy," *Nursing Research* 40 (1991): 69–75. The extent to which some of these symptoms are attributable to cocaine, as opposed to other drugs, is somewhat unclear because polydrug abuse is common among cocaine addicts.

47. American Medical Association Board of Trustees, "Legal Interventions during Pregnancy"; Dixon, "Effects of Transplacental Exposure."

48. Jeffrey A. Parness, "The Duty to Prevent Handicaps: Laws Promoting the Prevention of Handicaps to Newborns," *Western New England Law Review* 5 (1983): 431–64.

49. Chavkin, "Mandatory Treatment for Drug Use during Pregnancy"; American Medical Association Board of Trustees, "Legal Interventions during Pregnancy."

50. Wendy Chavkin, "Drug Addiction and Pregnancy: Policy Crossroads," *American Journal of Public Health* 80 (1990): 483–87; Walter B. Connolly, Jr., and Alison B. Marshall, "Drug Addiction, Pregnancy, and Childbirth: Legal Issues for the Medical and Social Services Communities," *Clinics in Perinatology* 18 (1991): 147–86.

51. Chavkin, "Mandatory Treatment for Drug Use during Pregnancy."

52. Some have suggested that postbirth prosecutions, as opposed to interventions during pregnancy, might be an appropriate response to pregnant women who abuse drugs or otherwise harm their offspring through culpable prenatal behavior. See Robertson, "Reconciling Offspring and Maternal Interests during Pregnancy." A number of authors have argued against postbirth sanctions, including Mary Anne Warren, "Women's Rights versus the Protection of Fetuses" in Fritz K. Beller and Robert F. Weir, eds., *The Beginning of Human Life* (Dordrecht: Kluwer Academic Publishers, 1994), 287–99. I agree that postbirth prosecutions are not an acceptable solution. However, to limit the length of my discussion, I shall not explore this topic.

53. Annas, "Forced Cesareans"; Annas, "Protecting the Liberty of Pregnant Patients," *New England Journal of Medicine* 316 (1987):1213–14; Kolder, Gallagher, and Parsons,

"Court-ordered Obstetrical Interventions"; Nelson and Milliken, "Compelled Medical Treatment"; Thomas L. Shriner, Jr., "Maternal Versus Fetal Rights — A Clinical Dilemma," *Obstetrics and Gynecology* 53 (1979): 518–19; Dawn E. Johnsen, "The Creation of Fetal Rights: Conflicts with Women's Constitutional Rights to Liberty, Privacy, and Equal Protection," *Yale Law Journal* 95 (1986): 599–625; Johnsen, "New Threat to Pregnant Women's Autonomy"; Nelson, Buggy, and Weil, "Forced Medical Treatment of Pregnant Women"; Fletcher, "Drawing Moral Lines"; Rhoden, "Judge in the Delivery Room"; Rhoden, "Cesareans and Samaritans"; Gallagher, "Prenatal Invasions and Interventions"; Gallagher, "Fetus as Patient"; Goldberg, "Medical Choices during Pregnancy"; Field, "Controlling the Woman to Protect the Fetus."

54. Annas, "Forced Cesareans"; Gallagher, "Prenatal Invasions and Interventions"; Johnsen, "New Threat to Pregnant Women's Autonomy."

55. *Jefferson v. Griffin Spalding County Hospital Authority* 274 S.E. 2d 457 (1981). Also, see the discussion of the Jeffries case in Poland, "Reproductive Technology and Responsibility," 71.

56. Kolder, Gallagher, and Parsons, "Court-ordered Obstetrical Interventions."

57. American Medical Association Board of Trustees, "Legal Interventions during Pregnancy."

58. American Academy of Pediatrics Committee on Bioethics, "Fetal Therapy: Ethical Considerations," *Pediatrics* 81 (1988): 898–99.

59. Frank A. Chervenak and Laurence B. McCullough, "Perinatal Ethics: A Practical Method of Analysis of Obligations to Mother and Fetus," *Obstetrics and Gynecology* 66 (1985): 442–46. In case it is claimed that I am not interpreting their view accurately, let us consider the reasons supporting this interpretation. In discussing maternal refusal of diagnostic procedures or treatment needed for the sake of the fetus, they stated:

> The following guidelines help to negotiate such a moral conflict. The greater the likelihood that a particular intervention will clearly result in a substantial benefit for the fetus, i.e., a significant decrease in morbidity and mortality, the stronger are the beneficence-based obligations to the fetus. The greater the likelihood that the fetus will be at substantial risk from the intervention, e.g., increased morbidity and mortality, the weaker are fetal beneficence-based obligations. The greater the risk of harm to the mother, i.e., increase in morbidity and mortality, the stronger are maternal autonomy-based obligations in those cases in which the woman refuses the intervention. These guidelines permit fetal diagnosis and treatment when the risks to the fetus are minimal, the potential benefit for the fetus is substantial, and the risks to the woman are those she should reasonably accept on behalf of her fetus.

The language of this statement seems plainly to assert that the three conditions in question are jointly sufficient for the ethical justifiability of coerced interventions. Other commentators have interpreted the passage in the same way (e.g., Nelson and Milliken, "Compelled Medical Treatment of Pregnant Women," p. 1064). Moreover, I put forward this interpretation in my article "Court-ordered Treatment in Obstetrics": "This view states, in effect, that morality should be legally enforced in the area of maternal treatment. Whenever the woman morally should consent to a procedure but refuses, the courts are ethically justified in forcing the procedure, provided the other conditions are satisfied" (p. 862). In their letter of the same title commenting on this article, Chervenak and McCullough did not disagree with this interpretation of their view. See *Obstetrics and Gynecology* 79 (1992): 476–77.

60. Chervenak and McCullough have acknowledged that there are such cases. See Frank A. Chervenak and Laurence B. McCullough, "Justified Limits on Refusing Intervention," *Hastings Center Report* 21 (1991): 12–18, where on p. 15 they state, "We have argued elsewhere that the pregnant woman, in a pregnancy being taken to term, is ethically obligated to accept reasonable risks on behalf of the fetus in the management of her pregnancy," citing their article "Perinatal Ethics."

61. Chervenak and McCullough, "Perinatal Ethics."

62. Chervenak, McCullough, and Skupski, "Ethical Justification for Emergency, Coerced Cesarean Delivery." The main points in that argument are the following. First, the pregnant woman and physician have beneficence-based obligations to protect the fetal patient and future child by preventing death and permanent central nervous system injury. Second, the clinical judgment that there is a significant risk of fetal death or permanent central nervous system damage that might be reduced by immediate cesarean delivery and might be increased by respecting refusal of cesarean section is well-founded and reliable. Third, provided the woman does not physically resist, the risks to her associated with cesarean delivery are extremely low and are risks she ought to take. From these three premises, Chervenak and McCullough conclude that it is ethically justifiable to perform cesarean section coercively, without a court order or the woman's consent, when the risks to her are minimal, which is true when she does not physically resist (see pp. 1032–33, esp. the summary of the argument on p. 1033.). However, there is a tremendous gap in this argument. As I pointed out above, the fact that the pregnant woman has an obligation to the fetus does not automatically justify coercing her to fulfill that obligation. Therefore, Chervenak and McCullough's assertion that the woman has obligations, while obviously true, does not by itself provide a solution in this case or any other case in which the woman is obligated to agree to treatment that would potentially provide a substantial net benefit to the fetal patient. What is needed is an argument that it is justifiable to enforce such obligations. Chervenak and McCullough provide no argument. They just state their conclusion that such obligations should be enforced. Thus, they fail to defend satisfactorily any of the following views: that coerced emergency cesarean section is ethically justifiable in this case; that coercive treatment is justifiable *whenever* the woman has an obligation to consent to treatment that is likely to provide a substantial net benefit to the fetal patient (as they claimed in the earlier article); or that coercive treatment is justifiable whenever the three premises stated above are satisfied.

63. Bowes and Selgestad, "Fetal versus Maternal Rights."

64. H. David Banta and Stephen B. Thacker, "Assessing the Costs and Benefits of Electronic Fetal Monitoring," *Obstetrical and Gynecological Survey* 34 (1979): 627–42.

65. Thus, the view of Chervenak and McCullough in question is both ethically and legally unjustifiable. Although they claimed that my arguments leading to this conclusion contained errors (Chervenak and McCullough, *Ethics in Obstetrics and Gynecology*, pp. 264–65, n. 39), I believe that I have adequately responded to these claims concerning supposed errors in nn. 26 and 35 above. In more recent work, Chervenak and

McCullough seem to abandon their earlier view. See "Justified Limits on Refusing Intervention"; *Ethics in Obstetrics and Gynecology,* pp. 245–65; "Court-ordered Cesarean Delivery" in Beller and Weir, *Beginning of Human Life,* 257–72. In these writings, they seem to put forward the view that coerced treatment is ethically justifiable in *some,* but not all, cases in which the woman ought to consent to treatment likely to provide substantial net benefit to the fetal patient. They focus on complete placenta previa and state that their conclusion that coerced cesarean sections are justifiable in that context are not to be applied automatically to other types of clinical situations. Here they are much more restrained in asserting that court orders are justifiable. On the face of it, they seem to have moved to a position that is much closer to the view I defended in "Court-ordered Treatment in Obstetrics." At one point they even state the following: ". . . that a pregnant woman has beneficence-based obligations to the fetal patient as its fiduciary does not mean that others, on this basis alone, have the moral authority to enforce that obligation" (*Ethics in Obstetrics and Gynecology,* p. 110).

Index

Toulmin, Stephen, 74, 207n2, 210n28
Trisomies *13* and *18,* 165–66, 229n45
Tubal ligation. *See* Sterilization
Twinning, 113, 127

Undue burden test, 31, 32
U.S. Supreme Court: on right to abortion, 30–32, 158, 164–66; on right to privacy, 28–32
Utilitarianism, 4, 66–68, 208nn10–11

Values, 2–3, 63–65, 159–62, 179–80; assigning priorities to, 63–81; conflicting, 3, 63

Vasectomy. *See* Sterilization
Vatican. *See* Roman Catholic church.
Veatch, Robert M., 69–72, 210n25
Viability: moral significance of, 49–53, 57; and U.S. Supreme Court, 164–66
Virtues, 65

Warren, Mary Ann, 55, 60–61
Whitehead, Mary Beth, 106
Whitehouse, Peter, 141–45
Wildes, Kevin Wm., 76

York v. Jones, 116–17